Official Journal of the

Collegium Internationale Allergologicum

CIA

International Archives of Allergy and Immunology

Founded 1950 by D. Harley, P. Kallós, W. Löffler and F.W. Wittich
Continued by E.A. Brown (1952–1954), W. Kaufman (1955–1967),
F. Hahn (1961–1972), H.C. Goodman (1963–1975),
R.R.A. Coombs (1955–1984), Z. Trnka (1972–1987), P. Kallós (1950–1988),
G.B. West (1959–1991), J. Bienenstock (1990–1991), L.Å. Hanson (1981–1991),
K. Kano (1982–1991), F. Milgrom (1965–1991), K. Rother (1982–1991),
G. Wick (1991–1997), B. Grubeck-Loebenstein (1991–1997), D. Kraft (1998–2002)

KARGER

Printed in Switzerland on acid-free and non-aging paper (ISO 9706) by Reinhardt Druck, Basel

Appears monthly: 3 volumes per year (12 issues)

Guidelines for Authors

International Archives of
Allergy and Immunology

'International Archives of Allergy and Immunology' appears monthly and provides a forum for publication of work from all aspects of modern allergology and immunology. Papers considered of special interest will be treated as 'hot topics' and every attempt will be made to publish these especially fast. The Editor-in-Chief, the Managing Editor and a team of internationally established Associate Editors competently covering all fields of allergology and immunology are responsible for the scientific quality of this international core journal. *International Archives* publishes original work in the fields of allergy, immunopathology and transplantation, cellular immunology, immunogenetics, immunopharmacology and immunoendocrinology, mucosal immunity, immunology of infectious diseases and immunology of connective tissue diseases. In addition, reviews, minireviews, commentaries and opinions on controversial subjects are published regularly. A new system of manuscript submission, reviewing and processing guarantees competent and fair reviewing as well as fast and high quality publication.

Submission

Only papers written in English are considered. Detailed Online Submission Instructions with a link to the Submission Website are at http://www.karger.com/iaa/. Before submitting your manuscript, you are encouraged to review the detailed guidelines at www.karger.com/iaa_guidelines for specific directions as how to get a manuscript ready for submission. If you should have any problems with your submission, or should you feel the need to submit the paper in a non-electronic form, please contact the editorial office:

S. Karger AG
Editorial Office 'International Archives of Allergy and Immunology'
PO Box
CH–4009 Basel (Switzerland)
Tel. +41 61 306 1360
Fax +41 61 306 1434
E-Mail e.lieberherr@karger.com

Mailing address for courier deliveries only:
Allschwilerstr. 10
CH–4055 Basel (Switzerland)

Original papers: Submitted manuscripts should be fully documented reports of original research. They must describe significant and original observations to be critically evaluated and, if necessary, repeated.

Short communications: These manuscripts should not contain more than ***2 printed pages (i.e. 6,460 characters per page),*** including an abstract, essential references and not more than 3 tables or figures. Such communications should represent complete, original studies and should be arranged in the same way as full-length manuscripts.

Novel Insights from Clinical Practice (formerly Case Reports): The publication space available for case reports is very limited. The journal only considers case reports with significant new insights or with an extremely unusual and memorable course. Highlighted boxes containing one or two bullet points on 'Established facts' (what is already known) and 'Novel insights' (what new information has been gained) are required and should be placed on the first page of the report. These should be selected so as to reinforce the novelty of the clinical observation. The manuscript should be presented with an abstract (unstructured, max. 200 words), followed by introduction, case report and discussion. Maximum 3 figures.

Review articles, minireviews, opinion articles, controversies and commentaries: Authors who wish to contribute a manuscript to one of these categories should contact the Editor-in-Chief. Minireviews should be focused, brief reports on topics of current interest. Commentaries should offer a more personalized perspective on a topic that will be of interest to the general readership. All contributions to these categories will be subject to Editorial review.

Letters to the Editor concerning work published in the journal may be submitted. They should not exceed 2 manuscript pages including one table or figure.

Conditions

All manuscripts are subject to editorial review. Manuscripts are received with the explicit understanding that they are not under simultaneous consideration by any other publication. A cover letter with the name, address, and telephone and telefax numbers of the corresponding author must accompany each manuscript. This letter must include a statement that affirms that all authors agree with the submission. Submission of an article for publication implies the transfer of the copyright from the author to the publisher upon acceptance. Accepted papers become the permanent property of *International Archives of Allergy and Immunology* and may not be reproduced by any means, in whole or in part, without the written consent of the publisher. It is the author's responsibility to obtain permission to reproduce illustrations, tables, etc. from other publications. One of the criteria considered in reviewing manuscripts is the proper treatment of animals. In particular, the use of painful or otherwise noxious stimuli must be carefully and thoroughly justified. Papers that do not meet these criteria will not be accepted for publication.

Conflict of Interest

Authors are required to disclose any sponsorship or funding arrangements, including that from companies, relating to their research. All authors should disclose any possible conflicts of interest in the cover letter to the editor and at the end of the article.

Plagiarism Policy

Whether intentional or not, plagiarism is a serious violation. We define plagiarism as a case in which a paper reproduces another work with at least 25% similarity and without citation.
If evidence of plagiarism is found before/after acceptance or after publication of the paper, the author will be offered a chance for rebuttal. If the arguments are not found to be satisfactory, the manuscript will be retracted and the author sanctioned from publishing papers for a period to be determined by the responsible Editor(s).

Arrangement

Manuscripts should be written in English and be as concise as possible.
Be sure to display line numbers (1, 2, 3, and so forth) in the left margin of the manuscript (line numbering can be added from the Page Setup or Format menu of word processing programs). The line numbering should be continuous throughout the entire manuscript, from the title page through to the final page (i.e., do not begin numbering from 1 again at the top of each page).

Title page: The first page of each paper should indicate a concise title, the authors' full names, affiliations and e-mail addresses, the institute where the work was conducted, and a short title for use as running head.

Full address: The exact postal address of the corresponding author complete with postal code must be given at the bottom of the title page. Please also supply phone and fax numbers, as well as an e-mail address.

Key words: Please supply 3–10 key words in English that reflect the content of the paper.

Abstract: **Provide on a separate page an abstract of not more than 250 words. This abstract should consist of four paragraphs, labeled Background, Methods, Results, and Conclusions. They should briefly describe, respectively, the problem being addressed in the study, how the study was performed, the salient results, and what the authors conclude from the results.**

The text should be arranged in the following sections: Introduction, Material and Methods, Results, Discussion, Acknowledgement, References.

Footnotes: Avoid footnotes. When essential, they are numbered consecutively and typed at the foot of the appropriate page.

Tables and illustrations: Tables and illustrations (both numbered in Arabic numerals) should be prepared on separate pages. Tables require a heading and figures a legend, also prepared on a separate page. For the reproduction of illustrations, only good drawings and original photographs can be accepted; negatives or photocopies cannot be used. Due to technical reasons, figures with a screen background should not be submitted. When possible, group several illustrations on one block for reproduction (max. size 180 × 223 mm) or provide crop marks. Each illustration must be labeled with its number and the author's name. Electronically submitted b/w half-tone and color illustrations must have a final resolution of 300 dpi after scaling (final size), line drawings one of 800–1,200 dpi. Figure files must not be embedded in a document file but submitted separately (see detailed instructions at www.karger.com/iaa/).

Color illustrations
Online edition: Color illustrations are reproduced free of charge. In the print version, the illustrations are reproduced in black and white. Please avoid referring to the colors in the text and figure legends.
Print edition: Up to 6 color illustrations per page can be integrated within the text at CHF 800.– per page.

Abbreviations: Avoid overuse of abbreviations. Introduce an abbreviation only when the same term occurs three or more times.

KARGER

E-Mail karger@karger.com
www.karger.com

The Guidelines for Authors are available at:
www.karger.com/iaa_Guidelines

References: In the text identify references by Arabic numerals [in square brackets]. Material submitted for publication but not yet accepted should be noted as 'unpublished data' and not be included in the reference list. The list of references should include only those publications which are cited in the text. Do not alphabetize; number references in the order in which they are first mentioned in the text. The surnames of the authors followed by initials should be given. There should be no punctuation other than a comma to separate the authors. Preferably, please cite all authors. Abbreviate journal names according to the Index Medicus system. Also see International Committee of Medical Journal Editors: Uniform requirements for manuscripts submitted to biomedical journals (www.icmje.org).

Examples
(a) Papers published in periodicals: Sun J, Koto H, Chung KF: Interaction of ozone and allergen challenges on bronchial responsiveness and inflammation in sensitised guinea pigs. Int Arch Allergy Immunol 1997;112:191–195.
(b) Papers published only with DOI numbers:
Theoharides TC, Boucher W, Spear K: Serum interleukin-6 reflects disease severity and osteoporosis in mastocytosis patients. Int Arch Allergy Immunol DOI: 10.1159/000063858.
(c) Monographs: Matthews DE, Farewell VT: Using and Understanding Medical Statistics, ed 3, revised. Basel, Karger, 1996.
(d) Edited books: Parren PWHI, Burton DR: Antibodies against HIV-1 from phage display libraries: Mapping of an immune response and progress towards antiviral immunotherapy; in Capra JD (ed): Antibody Engineering. Chem Immunol. Basel, Karger, 1997, vol 65, pp 18–56.

Full address: The exact postal address complete with postal code must be given at the bottom of the title page. Please also supply phone and fax numbers, as well as your e-mail address.

Reference Management Software: Use of EndNote® is recommended for easy management and formatting of citations and reference lists (format setting: *Intervirology*).

Digital Object Identifier (DOI)

S. Karger Publishers supports DOIs as unique identifiers for articles. A DOI number will be printed on the title page of each article. DOIs can be useful in the future for identifying and citing articles published online without volume or issue information. More information can be found at www.doi.org.

Supplementary Material

Supplementary material is restricted to additional data that are not necessary for the scientific integrity and conclusions of the paper. Please note that all supplementary files will undergo editorial review and should be submitted together with the original manuscript. The Editors reserve the right to limit the scope and length of the supplementary material. Supplementary material must meet production quality standards for Web publication without the need for any modification or editing. In general, supplementary files should not exceed 10 MB in size. All figures and tables should have titles and legends and all files should be supplied separately and named clearly. Acceptable files and formats are: Word or PDF files, Excel spreadsheets (only if the data cannot be converted properly to a PDF file), and video files (.mov, .avi, .mpeg).

Author's Choice™

Karger's Author's Choice™ service broadens the reach of your article and gives all users worldwide free and full access for reading, downloading and printing at www.Karger.com. The option is available for a one-time fee of CHF 3000.–, which is a permissible cost in grant allocation. More information can be found at www.karger.com/authors_choice.

NIH-Funded Research

The U.S. National Institutes of Health (NIH) mandates under the NIH Public Access Policy that final, peer-reviewed manuscripts appear in its digital database within 12 months of the official publication date. As a service to authors, Karger submits your manuscript on your behalf to PubMed Central (PMC) immediately upon publication. It usually receives a PMCID within approximately a month and will appear in PMC after 12 months. For those selecting our premium Author's ChoiceTM service, the usual embargo will be overridden, accelerating the accessibility of your work.

Self-Archiving

Karger permits authors to archive their pre-prints (i.e. pre-refereeing) or post-prints (i.e. final draft post-refereeing) on their personal or institution's servers, provided the following conditions are met: Articles may not be used for commercial purposes, must be linked to the publisher's version, and must acknowledge the publisher's copyright. Authors selecting Karger's Author's Choice™ feature, however, are also permitted to archive the final, published version of their article, which includes copyediting and design improvements as well as citation links.

Page Charges

There are no page charges for papers of 5 or fewer printed pages (including tables, illustrations and references). Each additional complete or partial page is charged to the author at CHF 325.–. The allotted size of a paper is 5 printed pages (6,460 characters per page), which is equal to approx. 14 manuscript pages including tables, illustrations and references.

Proofs

Unless indicated otherwise, proofs are sent to the corresponding author and should be returned with the least possible delay. Alterations other than the correction of printer's errors are charged to the author.

Reprints

Order forms and a price list are sent with the proofs. Orders submitted after the issue is printed are subject to considerably higher prices.

KARGER

E-Mail karger@karger.com
www.karger.com

The Guidelines for Authors are available at:
www.karger.com/iaa_Guidelines

General Information

International Archives of
Allergy and Immunology

ISSN Print Edition: 1018–2438
ISSN Online Edition: 1423–0097

Journal Homepage: www.karger.com/iaa

Publication Data: 'International Archives of Allergy and Immunology' is published 12 times a year. Volumes 160–162, each with 4 issues, appear in 2013.

Subscription Rates: Subscriptions run for a full calendar year. Prices are given per year.

Personal subscription:

Print or Online	Print+Online combined
CHF 172.–	CHF 316.–
EUR 139.–	EUR 256.–
USD 170.00	USD 314.00

postage and handling (added to print and print+online)
CHF 86.40 Europe, CHF 124.80 Overseas
EUR 67.20
USD 115.20

Institutional subscription:

Print or Online	Print+Online combined
CHF 5238.–	CHF 5763.–
EUR 4224.–	EUR 4647.–
USD 5187.00	USD 5706.00

postage and handling (added to print and print+online)
CHF 108.– Europe, CHF 156.– Overseas
EUR 84.–
USD 144.00

Airmail surcharge: CHF 105.– / USD 99.00

Back Volumes and Single Issues: Information on availability and prices of single print issues and print or electronic back volumes can be obtained from Customer Service at *service@karger.com.*

Bibliographic Indices: This journal is regularly listed in bibliographic services, including *Current Contents®* and PubMed/MEDLINE.

Photocopying: This journal has been registered with the Copyright Clearance Center (CCC), as indicated by the code appearing on the first page of each article. For readers in the US, this code signals consent for copying of articles for personal or internal use, or for the personal or internal use of specific clients, provided that the stated fee is paid per copy directly to
Copyright Clearance Center Inc.
222 Rosewood Drive
Danvers, MA 01923 (USA)
A copy of the first page of the article must accompany payment. Consent does not extend to copying for general distribution, for promotion, for creating new works, or for resale. In these cases, specific written permission must be obtained from the copyright owner,
S. Karger AG, P.O. Box
CH–4009 Basel (Switzerland).

Subscription Orders:
Orders can be placed at agencies, bookstores, directly with the Publisher

S. Karger AG
Medical and Scientific Publishers
Allschwilerstrasse 10
CH–4009 Basel
Switzerland

t: +41 61 306 11 11
f: +41 61 306 12 34
e: karger@karger.com
w: www.karger.com

(for courier services only:
Allschwilerstrasse 10
CH–4055 Basel)

or further Karger offices or representatives:

Germany
S. Karger GmbH
Postfach
79095 Freiburg
Deutschland
(Hausadresse: Wilhelmstrasse 20A, 79098 Freiburg)
t: +49 761 45 20 70
f: +49 761 45 20 714
e: information@karger.de
w: www.karger.de

Japan
Karger Japan, Inc.
Shiba Daimon Asahi Bldg. 2F
1-2-23 Shiba Daimon
Minato-ku
Tokyo 105-0012
Japan
t: +81 3 6435 6242
f: +81 3 6435 6244
e: publisher@karger.jp
w: www.karger.jp

USA
S. Karger Publishers, Inc.
26 West Avon Road
P.O. Box 529
Unionville, CT 06085
USA
Toll free: +1 800 828 5479
t: +1 860 675 7834
f: +1 860 675 7302
e: karger@snet.net

France
Librairie Médi-Sciences Sarl
36, bd de Latour-Maubourg
75007 Paris
France
t: +33 (0) 1 45 51 42 58
f: +33 (0) 1 45 56 07 80
e: librairie@medi-sciences.fr
w: www.medi-sciences.fr

South East Asia, China and Taiwan
Karger Regional Office (Malaysia)
CEO Suite Kuala Lumpur
Quill 7, 27th Floor
Jalan Stesen Sentral 5
KL Sentral
Kuala Lumpur 50470
Malaysia
t: +60 3 2776 6803
f: +60 3 2776 6999
e: service@karger.cn; r.chew@karger.cn

Karger China
10th Floor, Twin Towers (East)
B12 Jianguomenwai Avenue
Beijing 100022
China
t: +86 10 5123 5033
f: +86 10 5123 5122
e: service@karger.cn; r.chew@karger.cn
w: www.karger.cn

India, Bangladesh, Sri Lanka
Medscience India
Plot No. 17, Yusuf Sarai Market
B.L. Glass Building, 2nd Floor
Sri Aurobindo Marg
New Delhi 110 016
India
t: +91 11 46029 633
f: +91 11 46029 634
c: +91 98 91052 128
e: medsci.india@gmail.com

Change of Address:
Both old and new address should be sent to the subscription source.

KARGER

E-Mail karger@karger.com
www.karger.com

The Guidelines for Authors are available at:
www.karger.com/iaa_Guidelines

International Archives of
Allergy and
Immunology

Recent Advances in Hereditary Angioedema Self-Administration Treatment

Summary of an International Hereditary Angioedema Expert Meeting

Guest Editor
Timothy J. Craig, Hershey, Pa.

6 figures in color, and 13 tables, 2013

KARGER

Basel · Freiburg · Paris · London · New York · New Delhi · Bangkok · Beijing · Tokyo · Kuala Lumpur · Singapore · Sydney

Dr. Craig speaks for CSL Behring, ViroPharma, Shire and Dyax. He does research for Pharming, CSL Behring, ViroPharma, Shire and Dyax. He is a consultant for CSL Behring and Dyax and has received educational grants from Dyax, ViroPharma and CSL Behring.

The International Hereditary Angioedema Expert Meeting and this supplement were supported by CSL Behring.

S. Karger
Medical and Scientific Publishers
Basel · Freiburg · Paris · London · New York · New Delhi · Bangkok · Beijing · Tokyo · Kuala Lumpur · Singapore · Sydney

Disclaimer
The statements, opinions and data contained in this publication are solely those of the individual authors and contributors and not of the publisher and the editor(s). The appearance of advertisements in the journal is not a warranty, endorsement, or approval of the products or services advertised or of their effectiveness, quality or safety. The publisher and the editor(s) disclaim responsibility for any injury to persons or property resulting from any ideas, methods, instructions or products referred to in the content or advertisements.

Drug Dosage
The authors and the publisher have exerted every effort to ensure that drug selection and dosage set forth in this text are in accord with current recommendations and practice at the time of publication. However, in view of ongoing research, changes in government regulations, and the constant flow of information relating to drug therapy and drug reactions, the reader is urged to check the package insert for each drug for any change in indications and dosage and for added warnings and precautions. This is particularly important when the recommended agent is a new and/or infrequently employed drug.

Printed in Switzerland
on acid-free and non-aging paper (ISO 9706) by
Reinhardt Druck, Basel
ISBN 978–3–318–02430–2
e-ISBN 978–3–318–02431–9

KARGER

E-Mail karger@karger.com

Vol. 161, Suppl. 1, 2013

International Archives of
Allergy and
Immunology

Contents

KARGER

E-Mail karger@karger.com
www.karger.com/iaa

Foreword

International Archives of Allergy and Immunology

Int Arch Allergy Immunol 2013;161(suppl 1):1–2
DOI: 10.1159/000351228

Published online: May 28, 2013

Recent Advances in Hereditary Angioedema Self-Administration Treatment: Summary of an International Hereditary Angioedema Expert Meeting

Timothy J. Craig

College of Medicine, Penn State University, Hershey Medical Center, Hershey, Pa., USA

Overall Perspective

With more products becoming licensed for self-administration treatment of hereditary angioedema (HAE) [Berinert (C1 esterase inhibitor), Firazyr (icatibant) and Cinryze (C1 esterase inhibitor)] healthcare professionals are increasingly offering this option to their patients. To discuss issues relating to self-administration therapy of HAE, a group of experts from Europe, the USA and Canada met to share their experiences and to discuss how to encourage more patients to self-administer.

HAE is a rare autosomal dominant condition, with an estimated prevalence of between 1:10,000 and 1:50,000, which affects all ethnicities and age groups. Clinically, HAE is characterised by acute attacks of non-pitting, non-pruritic swelling of the skin and subcutaneous tissue and is potentially a life-threatening condition. To date, treatment approaches have included the management of acute attacks or prophylactic treatment. Recently, a number of therapies for self-administration have become licensed for use; however, self-administration has not been as widely adopted as one might have predicted.

This international HAE expert meeting, supported by an educational grant from CSL Behring, was held in Geneva, Switzerland, in June 2012. The aim of the meeting was to gain an insight into the current use of self-administration amongst patients from across Europe, the USA and Canada and to gain feedback on what needs to be done to encourage further use. This meeting enabled clinicians, nurses and a patient-expert to share their experience to date and to develop consensus of these experts in the field. The meeting highlighted differences between continents in the regulatory and legal frameworks for self-administration therapy and highlighted a need for further training resources for both healthcare teams and patients alike.

This supplement is divided into four papers which summarise the main points of consensus and areas that require further investigation to maximise the patient/physician experience. It was created following the international HAE expert meeting to highlight the need for further encouragement for the use of self-administration in order to improve patients' quality of life and to highlight areas for improvement to aid the management of treatment for patients. In the first article of this supplement, Cicardi et al. [1] highlight the current guidelines and published material on the treatment of HAE with particular consideration to the use of self-administration. The guidelines indicate the importance of training and follow-up and that self-administration may lead to an im-

KARGER

E-Mail karger@karger.com
www.karger.com/iaa

1018–2438/13/1615–0001$38.00/0

Correspondence to: Dr. Timothy J. Craig
College of Medicine, Penn State University
Hershey Medical Center
Hershey, PA 17033 (USA)
E-Mail tcraig@hmc.psu.edu

provement in patients' quality of life. In the second paper, by Caballero et al. [2], we report the feedback from a survey and participant experience with treating C1 esterase inhibitor deficiency. Data show a variety of experience throughout different clinics and that there are improvements that can be made to the current systems.

The practical aspects of self-administration are discussed in the third paper by Symons et al. [3], leading to the conclusions that patients are quick to learn the necessary skills, but further support such as a helpline would be a welcome addition to available resources. The final paper, by Boysen et al. [4], identifies some of the challenges faced by patients and that HAE awareness needs to be increased to improve patient diagnosis and treatment.

It is vital in today's changing medical field to take note of real-world clinical experience because it highlights potential areas for maximising further resources, development of best practice, removal of barriers, improved patient compliance and communication about therapy. We hope that information presented in this supplement will foster awareness of the benefits of self-administration and will raise awareness of HAE and its management.

I would like to express my thanks to all the participants of the international HAE expert meeting for their valuable contributions, and to CSL Behring for their support in the production of the supplement.

Disclosure Statement

Dr. Craig speaks for CSL Behring, ViroPharma, Shire and Dyax. He does research for Pharming, CSL Behring, ViroPharma, Shire and Dyax. He is a consultant for CSL Behring and Dyax and has received educational grants from Dyax, ViroPharma and CSL Behring.

References

1 Cicardi M, Craig TJ, Martinez-Saguer I, Hébert J, Longhurst HJ: Review of recent guidelines and consensus statements on hereditary angioedema therapy with focus on self-administration. Int Arch Allergy Immunol 2013;161(suppl 1):3–9.

2 Caballero T, Sala-Cunill A, Cancian M, Craig TJ, Neri S, Keith PK, Boccon-Gibod I, Bethune C, Bork K: Current status of implementation of self-administration training in various regions of Europe, Canada and the USA in the management of hereditary angioedema. Int Arch Allergy Immunol 2013;161 (suppl 1):10–16.

3 Symons C, Rossi O, Magerl M, Andritschke K: Practical approach to self-administration of intravenous C1-INH concentrate: a nursing perspective. Int Arch Allergy Immunol 2013; 161(suppl 1):17–20.

4 Boysen HB, Bouillet L, Aygören-Pürsün E: Challenges of C1-inhibitor concentrate self-administration. Int Arch Allergy Immunol 2013;161(suppl 1):21–25.

Review

International Archives of Allergy and Immunology

Int Arch Allergy Immunol 2013;161(suppl 1):3–9
DOI: 10.1159/000351232

Published online: May 28, 2013

Review of Recent Guidelines and Consensus Statements on Hereditary Angioedema Therapy with Focus on Self-Administration

M. Cicardi[a] T.J. Craig[b] I. Martinez-Saguer[c] J. Hébert[d] H.J. Longhurst[e]

[a]University of Milan and Luigi Sacco Hospital, Milan, Italy; [b]College of Medicine, Penn State University, Hershey Medical Center, Hershey, Pa., USA; [c]Johann Wolfgang Goethe-University Hospital, Frankfurt, Germany; [d]Laval University, Quebec, Que., Canada; [e]Barts Health NHS Trust, London, UK

Key Words
Hereditary angioedema · Self-administration · Consensus · Guidelines

Abstract
Consensus meetings and the resulting recommendations shape treatment choices in rare diseases such as hereditary angioedema (HAE) because they combine the experience of prescribing physicians and the patients who are receiving therapy. Self-administration of HAE therapy was recognised as a potential treatment option in the first consensus publication in 2003. Recent studies have confirmed that self-administration of therapy resolves attacks quickly, safely and minimises burden of disease; however, the discovery of inconsistent treatment approaches is a concern and warrants investigation into the barriers that prevent adherence with current recommendations.

Introduction

Recommended approaches to the treatment of hereditary angioedema (HAE) have been documented since 2003 when a consensus was reached on its diagnosis, therapy and management [1, 2]. Consensus meetings and the resulting recommendations shape treatment approaches in rare diseases where there is a paucity of clinical trials because they combine the valuable experience of prescribing physicians and the patients who are receiving therapy. Over recent years the results of phase III trials and observational studies have enhanced our understanding of HAE and consensus documents have been updated to reflect these developments. Most recently a global guideline, sponsored by the World Allergy Organization (WAO), was published in response to the consensus statements with the intent to standardise care for patients with HAE throughout the world [3]. Self-administration of HAE therapy was recognised as a potential treatment option in the first consensus document [1, 2] and has since been shown to be efficacious, safe and convenient [4]. Self-administration also offers the prospect of patients being able to manage symptoms while maintaining personal safety with minimal disruption in day-to-day life. The terminology used within the referenced material refers to both home therapy and self-administration. It is the understanding that home therapy/self-administration refers to treatment given in a non-healthcare setting by the patient, or a trained partner, outside of a healthcare facility. Here we review the development of consensus documents over time, focusing on self-administration of HAE treatment.

KARGER

E-Mail karger@karger.com
www.karger.com/iaa

1018–2438/13/1615–0003$38.00/0

Correspondence to: Prof. Marco Cicardi
Department of Biomedical and Clinical Sciences
University of Milan
Via G.B. Grassi, IT–20157 Milan (Italy)
E-Mail marco.cicardi@unimi.it

Ten Years of Developing Consensus Statements on HAE Therapy

In 2003, a meeting of representatives from European and North American centres was held in Canada, with the aim of developing a consensus algorithm. In this meeting it was recommended that home-care C1 esterase inhibitor (C1-INH) therapy be offered to patients with HAE and that these patients should be allowed to keep a supply of C1-INH replacement for personal use at home to be either self-administered or infused by a caregiver [2].

In 2005, a new consensus document was published [5] which supported the previous recommendation that all C1-INH-deficient patients should be offered the opportunity for home possession of C1-INH. Self-possession was shown to reduce the time patients spend awaiting infusion [6]. It was noted that patients should be allowed to keep sufficient therapeutic dose of C1-INH to treat a laryngeal attack, as 50–75% have a life-threatening attack at some time [7, 8]. It was advised that access to C1-INH for acute attacks should be optimised by home therapy training and that the management of patients who self-administer C1-INH concentrate should be standardised. Recommendations were made and are presented in table 1 [5].

In the 2005 guidelines, recommendations were made on the topics that home therapy training programmes should cover (table 2) [5]. In order for self-administration to be effective, a care management plan and good local transport links to an emergency department were deemed essential. It was also recommended that family physicians of self-administering patients be informed of their treatment choice [5].

In cases where the patient did not wish to, or was unable to self-administer C1-INH therapy, patients could keep a supply of concentrate for their use under the supervision of a health worker. This self-possession would reduce the time patients spend waiting for infusions. Consensus was that such a programme should be accompanied by appropriate information that should be carried by the patient for presentation at the emergency department in case of an attack and should include strategies for resupply of concentrate. It was also acknowledged that home possession may have benefits for children in the time to treatment from onset of attack [5].

In 2007, a review of studies detailing the use of C1-INH concentrate and home therapy in patients with HAE was published [9]. Patients who self-administered C1-INH (or had treatment infused by a family member), either on-demand at the onset of an attack or as regular prophylaxis, experienced improved quality of life and reduced severity, duration and frequency of attacks [10–15]. An excellent safety profile was also observed. At that time, children with HAE were still not usually considered for home therapy in the UK. One of the studies in this review used on-demand C1-INH therapy as first-line therapy for children, with regular prophylaxis for those who suffered frequent attacks; severe attacks were prevented and hospital time and absence from school were reduced [15]. The review concluded that the option of home therapy should potentially be made available to all HAE patients, adults and children, including those who suffer infrequent attacks [9].

The 2007 consensus document extended the idea of self-infusion and recommended that, for early treatment

Table 1. Recommendations for home therapy, 2005[a] [5]

Criteria for entry on to the home treatment programme
– Proven C1-INH deficiency.
– The patient's use of and compliance with prophylactic therapy should be optimal.
– In order to maintain required infusion skills, the patient should normally require infusion of C1-INH at least every 3 months.
– The patient must be motivated to comply with the home therapy programme and all its implications and be willing to be responsible for giving their home therapy. Written consent confirming this must be obtained before the programme is commenced.
– The patient must be counselled regarding the risk of transmissible infections from a blood product. The patient should demonstrate an understanding of this and provide written informed consent to receive therapy.
– The patient must have a partner willing to attend the home therapy programme who will be present when therapy is required.
– Written confirmation of support for home therapy must be agreed with the patient's general practitioner, including emergency support or an agreed pathway of emergency care.
– The patient must have access to a telephone when administering therapy.
– The patient must have good venous access.
– The patient must agree to call for an ambulance if self-cannulation is unsuccessful when concentrate is required.
– In most circumstances, home therapy is not employed in children.

[a] These guidelines have developed since 2005 and have progressed to now offer self-administration to all willing patients [25, 26, 40]. C1-INH = C1 esterase inhibitor.

Table 2. The home therapy training programme, 2005 [5]

The home therapy training programme should include the following key topics:

- Appropriate use of concentrate.
- Hand washing and aseptic technique.
- Supply and storage of concentrate and equipment.
- Preparation of equipment for administration of concentrate.
- Product checking procedure, i.e. dosage, expiry date.
- Demonstration of correct technique for reconstitution of solution.
- Cannulation with butterfly.
- Blood sampling pre-injection/infusion.
- Administration of injection/management of infusion.
- Management of adverse reactions.
- Automatically injectable adrenaline/epinephrine training (for treatment of anaphylaxis of infusion).
- Disposal of equipment.
- Documentation, e.g. accurate recording of batch number.
- Documentary evidence of the individual's training and competence.
- Receiving and monitoring infusion logs and other relevant documentation for any indication of difficulties.
- Investigating any adverse reactions/events and taking appropriate action.
- Keeping the specialist nurse/consultant immunologist informed of any relevant issues regarding care and treatment.
- Compliance with clinic visits.
- Performing an annual review of the individual's competence to administer injection/infusion.
- Liaising with the individual, his/her general practitioner, consultant immunologist and other relevant care providers.

of acute HAE attacks (and to facilitate prophylaxis where necessary), home C1-INH replacement self-infusion programmes should be offered to patients. These programmes are similar to the haemophilia self-infusion protocols which have been in use for over three decades [16]. The consensus meeting recommended that home self-infusion protocols should be available on patient websites and proposed the establishment of Comprehensive Care Clinics for the diagnosis, therapy and management of HAE, including the development of home infusion and home-care programmes. Comprehensive Care Clinics should be encouraged to register HAE patients in national and international database registries to facilitate research into the diagnosis and management of this disorder [17].

Although C1-INH (namely Berinert) has been approved in Germany for the treatment of acute HAE attacks since 1979 [18], C1-INH was only available on an individual 'compassionate use' basis in other parts of Europe and only became available in the USA in the latter part of the last decade: Berinert was approved for the treatment of acute HAE attacks in 23 European countries in 2008 [19] and in the USA in 2009 [20]; Cinryze was approved by the Food and Drug Administration (FDA) for routine prophylaxis in 2008 [21] and for self-administration for prophylaxis in 2009 [22]. Around this time, two new products were licensed for the treatment of acute HAE attacks: ecallantide (Kalbitor, a kallikrein inhibitor) was licensed in the USA [23] and icatibant (Firazyr, a bradykinin β_2-receptor) was licensed in Europe [24].

In 2009, the HAE international home therapy consensus document was formulated [25]. Initially, most self-administered treatment was limited to pasteurised-nanofiltered C1-INH replacement. It was agreed that every patient with HAE should be considered for self-administration training, once the diagnosis of C1-INH deficiency was confirmed. Extremes of age were no longer seen as a limiting factor in self-administration, although children needed a responsible adult willing to undertake training. It was strongly recommended that patients train with a 'home therapy partner' who would be able to provide support, advice and, where applicable, be trained to administer therapy. In the absence of a 'home therapy partner', it was recommended that extra care be taken with arrangements for medical back-up. Home therapy was recommended in pregnant and lactating women. It was stated that attacks at all sites could be self-treated; however, in the case of laryngeal oedema, patients should be urgently transferred to hospital after home therapy. Self-administration was found to be associated with a low incidence of 'cannulation failure' and could preserve veins more effectively than hospital-based care [25].

The consensus view was that the self-infusion training programme should be conducted over several sessions to ensure that the patient and treatment partner have sufficient practice to be familiar and confident with technical and medical aspects of self-administration. Prior to starting home therapy, the patient should have received the proposed home therapy at least once and have self-administered the therapy under medical supervision. The patient's and treatment partner's knowledge should be assessed upon completion of training and refresher training planned at least every 12 months [25]. Furthermore, it was noted that there was a need to optimise prophylaxis but home therapy need not be delayed since training can take place simultaneously with other treatments, and in most patients, attacks occur despite prophylaxis [25].

The 2010 international consensus algorithm for the diagnosis, therapy and management of HAE [26] agreed with the 2007 consensus document that home pasteurised-nanofiltered C1-INH self-infusion programmes should be offered to patients and be similar to haemophilia self-infusion programmes. It was also recommended that HAE patients be linked to a Comprehensive Care Clinic which must provide accountability for home- and hospital-based use of potentially toxic treatments, track patient outcomes and develop and meet Standards of Care for HAE. Comprehensive Care Clinic programmes should combine clinical care, education and research, and provide hospital-based patients with education of and accessibility to home therapy programmes.

Shortly after the release of these consensus documents, several phase III trials and other studies were reported [27–32] and the recommendations were updated to state that HAE patients should carry two doses of any of the HAE therapies. With the availability of newer treatments, the two doses could be plasma-derived C1-INH, recombinant human C1-INH, icatibant or ecallantide [33].

In 2011, Cinryze was granted European marketing authorisation for self-administration for routine prevention and treatment of acute HAE attacks in adults and adolescents [34]; also in 2011, Firazyr was approved by the FDA [35] and in Europe [36], and Berinert was approved in Europe [37] for self-administration of treatment for acute attacks. In 2012, Berinert was approved for self-administration for acute attacks in the USA [38]. Recently, Berinert was approved for short-term prophylaxis in Europe [39].

In 2012, evidence-based recommendations for the management of HAE were published by the Hereditary Angioedema International Working Group (HAWK) [40]. This consensus stated that all patients with HAE should have access to at least one therapy out of plasma-derived C1-INH, recombinant C1-INH, icatibant and ecallantide. Additionally, wherever possible, and permitted by specific prescribing guidelines, patients should have the on-demand medicine to treat acute attacks at home and should be trained to self-administer these agents. This recommendation was based on observations that greater efficacy of early on-demand treatment was reported compared with hospital therapy [14, 41]. This consensus document concluded that further investigation is needed to determine whether implementation of aggressive early home on-demand treatment would reduce the need for prophylactic treatment in patients whose attacks are insufficiently controlled by standard on-demand treatment, and that a more proactive, patient-centric approach towards HAE treatment needs to be implemented [40].

Finally, the WAO global guideline for HAE also endorsed self-care and home care of HAE by both consensus and evidence-based medicine [3]. The guideline was approved by the affiliated Allergy Immunology Associations worldwide. It emphasised that all therapies should be available to all patients with HAE worldwide and that home- and self-administration are preferred since they reduce morbidity, absenteeism, cost, disease burden and potential mortality, and improve quality of life.

Consensus on Home Therapy in Children and Adolescents

A consensus on therapeutic strategies in children and adolescents with HAE has recently been published. It concludes that home therapy with pasteurised-nanofiltered C1-INH is possible for trained and educated patients (or their parents or guardians) and that a home therapy regimen is reasonable when long-term prophylaxis is necessary; however, the frequency of attacks appropriate for this therapeutic option needs to be defined [42].

Current HAE Treatment Options

Currently there are two HAE treatment strategies licensed for self-administration: pasteurised-nanofiltered C1-INH and icatibant [4]. Several studies of self-administered HAE therapy have been published (table 3) and they confirm that self-administration of HAE therapy resolves attacks quickly and safely, and gives patients greater confidence in managing their condition. General consensus is such that self-administration should be offered to patients whenever possible.

Compliance with Current Treatment Recommendations

Consensus documents have been in circulation for almost a decade; however, a web-based survey in the USA conducted between October 2009 and February 2010 (at a similar time to the FDA approval of pasteurised-nanofiltered C1-INH), found that although more than 90% of the 172 responding physicians recommended treating acute HAE attacks, only half of them had used C1-INH to do so and very few had patients who self-treated (8.1%)

Table 3. Recent studies detailing home therapy in patients with HAE

Author	Year	Therapy	Outcome
Kreuz et al. [41]	2009	Regular doses of pasteurised-nanofiltered C1-INH	Completely abolished incidence of laryngeal oedema and reduced incidence of acute attacks.
Tourangeau et al. [43]	2012	On-demand C1-INH in clinic or home setting	Significant decreases in attack duration, pain medication use and graded attack severity in home setting vs. clinic.
Kreuz et al. [44]	2012	Paediatrics, previously on physician-based therapy switched to C1-INH as on-demand or individual replacement therapy	Decreased mean annual number of days hospitalised, time from onset of attack to administration of C1-INH and median time to initial symptom relief with home- vs. physician-based therapy.
Bygum et al. [45]	2009	Self-administered C1-INH	Self-administration of C1-INH improved quality of life on both physical and psychological parameters.
Farkas et al. [46]	2012	Icatibant administered by healthcare providers for home treatment of attacks[a]	All attacks resolved and safety was consistent with known local tolerability profile of icatibant.
Boccon-Gibod et al. [47]	2012	Self-administered icatibant	Complete symptom resolution. Patients felt greater confidence in managing their condition.

[a] At the time of this study, icatibant was licensed for administration by healthcare providers only; it is now licensed for self-administration. C1-INH = C1 esterase inhibitor; HAE = hereditary angioedema.

or received home healthcare assistance (3.5%) [48]. Furthermore, a recent survey (conducted between November 2010 and February 2011) showed that many international physicians neither adhere to the 2010 International Consensus Algorithm for treating HAE nor follow current evidence-based studies [49]; however, until recently, some physicians have been unable to adhere to such guidelines because of lack of approval of HAE treatments in their countries [48]. Since the US survey, clinical experience has increased significantly and this should help to improve compliance with current treatment recommendations. For example, in Frankfurt University Hospital, where C1-INH therapy has been available for many years, 74% of patients with HAE receive on-demand C1-INH therapy, 49% of patients are self-administering their therapy and treatment is individualised to limit disruption to normal daily activities [18].

These inconsistent treatment approaches are a concern and warrant investigation into potential barriers that prevent adherence with current recommendations. Emphasis should be placed on the education of physicians and nurses to raise their awareness of, and compliance with current HAE treatment recommendations. Patients should also be encouraged to take a proactive role in the management of their condition.

Conclusion

In summary, consensus group meetings have recommended that self-administration and self-possession of treatment are beneficial to patients with HAE. Recent studies have confirmed this showing that acute attacks are resolved quickly and safely with self-treatment, minimising the burden of disease. To date, guidelines essentially see only pasteurised-nanofiltered C1-INH and icatibant as real self-administration opportunities; however, ecallantide is approved for home-administration by a healthcare provider in the USA. Resources need to be maximised to encourage more patients to move to self-administration and to increase physicians' awareness of treatment recommendations.

Disclosure Statement

Professor Cicardi has a consultancy agreement with Sigma Tau and has been involved in advisory boards for CSL Behring, Dyax, ViroPharma and Sobi.

Dr. Craig speaks for CSL Behring, ViroPharma, Shire and Dyax. He does research for Pharming, CSL Behring, ViroPharma, Shire and Dyax. He is a consultant for CSL Behring and Dyax and has received educational grants from Dyax, ViroPharma and CSL Behring.

Dr. Martinez-Saguer gives lectures or is a consultant for the following companies: Bayer, Baxter, CSL Behring, Jerini/shire, Octapharma and Sobi.

Dr. Hébert is a consultant for GSK, Novartis, Merck, Paladin, Pfizer and Hollister Stier, and does clinical research for Circassia, BI, GSK, Merck, Novartis, AstraZeneca, Shire, Janssen and Pfizer.

Dr. Longhurst and members of her department have received funding to attend conferences and other educational events, have acted as medical advisors or speakers, have received donations to her departmental fund, have received financial and other assistance with patient care projects and/or have participated in clinical trials with the following companies: CSL Behring, Pharming/Swedish Orphan Biovitrum, Jerini/Shire, Dyax, ViroPharma, Baxter and Grifols.

References

1 Bowen T, Hebert J, Ritchie B, Burnham J, MacSween M, Warrington R, Yang W, Issekutz A, Karitsiotis N, McCombie N, Giulivi T: Management of hereditary angioedema: a Canadian approach. Transfus Apher Sci 2003; 29:205–214.

2 Bowen T, Cicardi M, Farkas H, Bork K, Kreuz W, Zingale L, Varga L, Martinez-Saguer I, Aygören-Pürsün E, Binkley K, Zuraw B, Davis A 3rd, Hebert J, Ritchie B, Burnham J, Castaldo A, Menendez A, Nagy I, Harmat G, Bucher C, Lacuesta G, Issekutz A, Warrington R, Yang W, Dean J, Kanani A, Stark D, McCusker C, Wagner E, Rivard GE, Leith E, Tsai E, MacSween M, Lyanga J, Serushago B, Leznoff A, Waserman S, de Serres J: Canadian 2003 International Consensus Algorithm for the Diagnosis, Therapy, and Management of Hereditary Angioedema. J Allergy Clin Immunol 2004;114:629–637.

3 Craig T, Aygören-Pürsün E, Bork K, Bowen T, Boysen H, Farkas H, Grumach A, Katelaris CH, Lockey R, Longhurst H, Lumry W, Magerl M, Martinez-Saguer I, Ritchie B, Nast A, Pawankar R, Zuraw B, Maurer M: WAO Guideline for the Management of Hereditary Angioedema. World Allergy Organ J 2012;5: 182–199.

4 Bork K: Current management options for hereditary angioedema. Curr Allergy Asthma Rep 2012;12:273–280.

5 Gompels MM, Lock RJ, Abinun M, Bethune CA, Davies G, Grattan C, Fay AC, Longhurst HJ, Morrison L, Price A, Price M, Watters D: C1 inhibitor deficiency: consensus document. Clin Exp Immunol 2005;139:379–394.

6 Agostoni A, Aygören-Pürsün E, Binkley KE, Blanch A, Bork K, Bouillet L, Bucher C, Castaldo AJ, Cicardi M, Davis AE, De Carolis C, Drouet C, Duponchel C, Farkas H, Fáy K, Fekete B, Fischer B, Fontana L, Füst G, Giacomelli R, Gröner A, Hack CE, Harmat G, Jakenfelds J, Juers M, Kalmár L, Kaposi PN, Karádi I, Kitzinger A, Kollár T, Kreuz W, Lakatos P, Longhurst HJ, Lopez-Trascasa M, Martinez-Saguer I, Monnier N, Nagy I, Németh E, Nielsen EW, Nuijens JH, O'Grady C, Pappalardo E, Penna V, Perricone C, Perricone R, Rauch U, Roche O, Rusicke E, Späth PJ, Szendei G, Takács E, Tordai A, Truedsson L, Varga L, Visy B, Williams K, Zanichelli A, Zingale L: Hereditary and acquired angioedema: problems and progress: proceedings of the third C1 esterase inhibitor deficiency workshop and beyond. J Allergy Clin Immunol 2004;114:S51–S131.

7 Bork K, Hardt J, Schicketanz KH, Ressel N: Clinical studies of sudden upper airway obstruction in patients with hereditary angioedema due to C1 esterase inhibitor deficiency. Arch Intern Med 2003;163:1229–1235.

8 Cicardi M, Bergamaschini L, Marasini B, Boccassini G, Tucci A, Agostoni A: Hereditary angioedema: an appraisal of 104 cases. Am J Med Sci 1982;284:2–9.

9 Longhurst HJ, Carr S, Khair K: C1-inhibitor concentrate home therapy for hereditary angioedema: a viable, effective treatment option. Clin Exp Immunol 2007;147:11–17.

10 Bork K, Meng G, Staubach P, Hardt J: Treatment with C1 inhibitor concentrate in abdominal pain attacks of patients with hereditary angioedema. Transfusion 2005;45:1774–1784.

11 Bork K, Witzke G: Long-term prophylaxis with C1-inhibitor (C1 INH) concentrate in patients with recurrent angioedema caused by hereditary and acquired C1-inhibitor deficiency. J Allergy Clin Immunol 1989;83:677–682.

12 Kreuz W, Fischer D, Martinez-Saguer I, Heller C, Klarmann D: C1-esterase inhibitor substitution in hereditary angioedema. Biomed Prog 1999;12:1–7.

13 Kreuz W, Martinez-Saguer I, Aygören-Pürsün E, Rusicke E, Klingebiel T: Individual replacement therapy (IRT) with a pasteurized C1-inhibitor concentrate compared to prophylaxis with danazol in patients with hereditary angioedema (HAE) – a prospective study. Blood 2004;104:1028 (abstract).

14 Levi M, Choi G, Picavet C, Hack CE: Self-administration of C1-inhibitor concentrate in patients with hereditary or acquired angioedema caused by C1-inhibitor deficiency. J Allergy Clin Immunol 2006;117:904–908.

15 Rusicke E, Martinez-Saguer I, Aygören-Pürsün E, Kreuz W: Home treatment in patients with hereditary angioedema (HAE). J Allergy Clin Immunol 2006;117:S180.

16 Strawczynski H, Stachewitsch A, Morgenstern G, Shaw ME: Delivery of care to hemophiliac children: home care versus hospitalization. Pediatrics 1973;51:986–991.

17 Bowen T, Cicardi M, Bork K, Zuraw B, Frank M, Ritchie B, Farkas H, Varga L, Zingale LC, Binkley K, Wagner E, Adomaitis P, Brosz K, Burnham J, Warrington R, Kalicinsky C, Mace S, McCusker C, Schellenberg R, Celeste L, Hebert J, Valentine K, Poon MC, Serushago B, Neurath D, Yang W, Lacuesta G, Issekutz A, Hamed A, Kamra P, Dean J, Kanani A, Stark D, Rivard GE, Leith E, Tsai E, Waserman S, Keith PK, Page D, Marchesin S, Longhurst HJ, Kreuz W, Rusicke E, Martinez-Saguer I, Aygören-Pürsün E, Harmat G, Füst G, Li H, Bouillet L, Caballero T, Moldovan D, Späth PJ, Smith-Foltz S, Nagy I, Nielsen EW, Bucher C, Nordenfelt P, Xiang ZY: Hereditary angiodema: a current state-of-the-art review, VII: Canadian Hungarian 2007 International Consensus Algorithm for the Diagnosis, Therapy, and Management of Hereditary Angioedema. Ann Allergy Asthma Immunol 2008;100:S30–S40.

18 Aygören-Pürsün E, Martinez-Saguer I, Rusicke E, Klingebiel T, Kreuz W: On demand treatment and home therapy of hereditary angioedema in Germany – the Frankfurt experience. Allergy Asthma Clin Immunol 2010;6:21.

19 CSL Behring: CSL Behring announces completion of national marketing authorizations of Berinert® after MRP in 23 European countries. 2011. http://www.cslbehring.com/PRelease/Berinert-Approved.htm?tabSelections=1255923338674&currentPage=1 (accessed 21 November 2012).

20 Food and Drug Administration: FDA approves Berinert to treat abdominal attacks, facial swelling associated with hereditary angioedema. 2009. http://www.fda.gov/NewsEvents/Newsroom/PressAnnouncements/2009/ucm186257.htm (accessed 21 November 2012).

21 Food and Drug Adminstration: Cinryze approval. 2008. http://www.fda.gov/BiologicsBloodVaccines/BloodBloodProducts/ApprovedProducts/LicensedProductsBLAs/FractionatedPlasmaProducts/ucm150480.htm (accessed 21 November 2012).

22 ViroPharma Inc.: ViroPharma receives complete response letter for Cinryze™ supplemental biologics licence application for acute treatment of hereditary angioedema. 2009. http://ir.viropharma.com/releasedetail.cfm?ReleaseID=543136 (accessed 21 November 2012).

23 Waknine Y: FDA approves ecallantide for hereditary angioedema. 2009. http://www.medscape.com/viewarticle/713401 (accessed 21 November 2012).
24 Shire: Jerini receives European Commission approval for Firazyr (icatibant) in the treatment of HAE. 2008. http://www.shire.com/shireplc/en/media/shirenews?year=2008 (accessed 21 November 2012).
25 Longhurst HJ, Farkas H, Craig T, Aygören-Pürsün E, Bethune C, Bjorkander J, Bork K, Bouillet L, Boysen H, Bygum A, Caballero T, Cicardi M, Dempster J, Gompels M, Gooi J, Grigoriadou S, Huffer U, Kreuz W, Levi MM, Long J, Martinez-Saguer I, Raguet M, Reshef A, Bowen T, Zuraw B: HAE international home therapy consensus document. Allergy Asthma Clin Immunol 2010;6:22.
26 Bowen T, Cicardi M, Farkas H, Bork K, Longhurst HJ, Zuraw B, Aygoeren-Pürsün E, Craig T, Binkley K, Hebert J, Ritchie B, Bouillet L, Betschel S, Cogar D, Dean J, Devaraj R, Hamed A, Kamra P, Keith PK, Lacuesta G, Leith E, Lyons H, Mace S, Mako B, Neurath D, Poon MC, Rivard GE, Schellenberg R, Rowan D, Rowe A, Stark D, Sur S, Tsai E, Warrington R, Waserman S, Ameratunga R, Bernstein J, Björkander J, Brosz K, Brosz J, Bygum A, Caballero T, Frank M, Fust G, Harmat G, Kanani A, Kreuz W, Levi M, Li H, Martinez-Saguer I, Moldovan D, Nagy I, Nielsen EW, Nordenfelt P, Reshef A, Rusicke E, Smith-Foltz S, Späth P, Varga L, Xiang ZY: 2010 International consensus algorithm for the diagnosis, therapy and management of hereditary angioedema. Allergy Asthma Clin Immunol 2010;6:24.
27 Zuraw BL, Busse PJ, White M, Jacobs J, Lumry W, Baker J, Craig T, Grant JA, Hurewitz D, Bielory L, Cartwright WE, Koleilat M, Ryan W, Schaefer O, Manning M, Patel P, Bernstein JA, Friedman RA, Wilkinson R, Tanner D, Kohler G, Gunther G, Levy R, McClellan J, Redhead J, Guss D, Heyman E, Blumenstein BA, Kalfus I, Frank MM: Nanofiltered C1 inhibitor concentrate for treatment of hereditary angioedema. N Engl J Med 2010;363: 513–522.
28 Zuraw B, Cicardi M, Levy RJ, Nuijens JH, Relan A, Visscher S, Haase G, Kaufman L, Hack CE: Recombinant human C1-inhibitor for the treatment of acute angioedema attacks in patients with hereditary angioedema. J Allergy Clin Immunol 2010;126:821–827.
29 Cicardi M, Banerji A, Bracho F, Malbrán A, Rosenkranz B, Riedl M, Bork K, Lumry W, Aberer W, Bier H, Bas M, Greve J, Hoffmann TK, Farkas H, Reshef A, Ritchie B, Yang W, Grabbe J, Kivity S, Kreuz W, Levy RJ, Luger T, Obtulowicz K, Schmid-Grendelmeier P, Bull C, Sitkauskiene B, Smith WB, Toubi E, Werner S, Anné S, Björkander J, Bouillet L, Cillari E, Hurewitz D, Jacobson KW, Katelaris CH, Maurer M, Merk H, Bernstein JA, Feighery C, Floccard B, Gleich G, Hébert J, Kaatz M, Keith P, Kirkpatrick CH, Langton D, Martin L, Pichler C, Resnick D, Wombolt D, Fernández Romero DS, Zanichelli A, Arcoleo F, Knolle J, Kravec I, Dong L, Zimmermann J, Rosen K, Fan WT: Icatibant, a new bradykinin-receptor antagonist, in hereditary angioedema. N Engl J Med 2010;363:532–541.
30 Cicardi M, Levy RJ, McNeil DL, Li HH, Sheffer AL, Campion M, Horn PT, Pullman WE: Ecallantide for the treatment of acute attacks in hereditary angioedema. N Engl J Med 2010; 363:523–531.
31 Levy RJ, Lumry WR, McNeil DL, Li HH, Campion M, Horn PT, Pullman WE: EDEMA4: a phase 3, double-blind study of subcutaneous ecallantide treatment for acute attacks of hereditary angioedema. Ann Allergy Asthma Immunol 2010;104:523–529.
32 Craig TJ, Levy RJ, Wasserman RL, Bewtra AK, Hurewitz D, Obtulowicz K, Reshef A, Ritchie B, Moldovan D, Shirov T, Grivcheva-Panovska V, Kiessling PC, Keinecke HO, Bernstein JA: Efficacy of human C1 esterase inhibitor concentrate compared with placebo in acute hereditary angioedema attacks. J Allergy Clin Immunol 2009;124:801–808.
33 Bowen T: Hereditary angioedema: beyond international consensus – circa December 2010 – The Canadian Society of Allergy and Clinical Immunology Dr. David McCourtie Lecture. Allergy Asthma Clin Immunol 2011;7:1.
34 ViroPharma Inc.: ViroPharma's Cinryze® (C1 inhibitor [human]) granted European marketing authorization for hereditary angioedema (HAE). 2011. http://ir.viropharma.com/releasedetail.cfm?ReleaseID=585060 (accessed 21 November 2012).
35 Shire: FDA approves Shire's Firazyr (icatibant injection) for acute attacks of hereditary angioedema (HAE). 2011. http://www.shire.com/shireplc/en/media/shirenews?id=520 (accessed 21 November 2012).
36 European Commission approves self-administration label for Firazyr® (icatibant) for the symptomatic treatment of acute hereditary angioedema attacks. 2011. http://www.pharmiweb.com/PressReleases/pressrel.asp?ROW_ID=37878#axzz2Cm0UVl3D (accessed 21 November 2012).
37 CSL Behring: CSL Behring receives European Health Authorities' approval for self-administration of Berinert®. 2011. http://www.cslbehring.com/news-room/european-health-authorities-approve-self-adminstration-of-berinert.htm (accessed 21 November 2012).
38 CSL Behring: CSL Behring receives FDA approval of expanded label on Berinert® for self-administration and treatment of acute laryngeal attacks of hereditary angioedema. 2012. http://www.cslbehring-us.com/news-room/HAE-Berinert-Self-Administration-and-Laryngeal-Attacks (accessed 21 November 2012).
39 CSL Behring: CSL Behring receives European Health Authorities' approval of Berinert® for short-term prophylaxis in adults and children. 2013. http://www.cslbehring.com/s1/cs/enco/1151517263302/news/1255931201677/prdetail.htm (accessed 17 April 2013).
40 Cicardi M, Bork K, Caballero T, Craig T, Li HH, Longhurst H, Reshef A, Zuraw B, HAWK: Evidence-based recommendations for the therapeutic management of angioedema owing to hereditary C1 inhibitor deficiency: consensus report of an International Working Group. Allergy 2012;67:147–157.
41 Kreuz W, Martinez-Saguer I, Aygören-Pürsün E, Rusicke E, Heller C, Klingebiel T: C1-inhibitor concentrate for individual replacement therapy in patients with severe hereditary angioedema refractory to danazol prophylaxis. Transfusion 2009;49:1987–1995.
42 Wahn V, Aberer W, Eberl W, Fasshauer M, Kühne T, Kurnik K, Magerl M, Meyer-Olson D, Martinez-Saguer I, Späth P, Staubach-Renz P, Kreuz W: Hereditary angioedema (HAE) in children and adolescents-a consensus on therapeutic strategies. Eur J Pediatr 2012;171:1339–1348.
43 Tourangeau LM, Castaldo AJ, Davis DK, Koziol J, Christiansen SC, Zuraw BL: Safety and efficacy of physician-supervised self-managed C1 inhibitor replacement therapy. Int Arch Allergy Immunol 2012;157:417–424.
44 Kreuz W, Rusicke E, Martinez-Saguer I, Aygören-Pürsün E, Heller C, Klingebiel T: Home therapy with intravenous human C1-inhibitor in children and adolescents with hereditary angioedema. Transfusion 2012;52: 100–107.
45 Bygum A, Andersen KE, Mikkelsen CS: Self-administration of intravenous C1-inhibitor therapy for hereditary angioedema and associated quality of life benefits. Eur J Dermatol 2009;19:147–151.
46 Farkas H, Csuka D, Zotter Z, Varga L, Böröcz Z, Temesszentandrási G, Jakab L, Karádi I: Home treatment of hereditary angioedema with icatibant administered by health care professionals. J Allergy Clin Immunol 2012; 129:851–852.
47 Boccon-Gibod I, Bouillet L: Safety and efficacy of icatibant self-administration for acute hereditary angioedema. Clin Exp Immunol 2012;168:303–307.
48 Riedl M: Hereditary angioedema therapies in the United States: movement toward an international treatment consensus. Clin Ther 2012;34:623–630.
49 Dispenza MC, Craig TJ: Discrepancies between guidelines and international practice in treatment of hereditary angioedema. Allergy Asthma Proc 2012;33:241–248.

Original Paper

International Archives of Allergy and Immunology

Int Arch Allergy Immunol 2013;161(suppl 1):10–16
DOI: 10.1159/000351233

Published online: May 28, 2013

Current Status of Implementation of Self-Administration Training in Various Regions of Europe, Canada and the USA in the Management of Hereditary Angioedema

T. Caballero[a] A. Sala-Cunill[b] M. Cancian[c] T.J. Craig[e] S. Neri[d] P.K. Keith[f] I. Boccon-Gibod[g] C. Bethune[h] K. Bork[i]

[a]Hospital La Paz Institute for Health Research (IdiPaz), Madrid, and [b]University of Barcelona, Barcelona, Spain; [c]University of Padova, Padova, and [d]University of Catania, Catania, Italy; [e]College of Medicine, Penn State University, Hershey Medical Center, Hershey, Pa., USA; [f]McMaster University, Hamilton, Ont., Canada; [g]National Reference Center for Angioedema, Internal Medicine Department, Grenoble University Hospital, Grenoble, France; [h]Derriford Hospital, Plymouth, UK; [i]Johannes Gutenberg University, Mainz, Germany

Key Words
Hereditary angioedema · Self-administration · Current status · Benefits · Quality of life

Abstract
Results from a 16-question survey about self-administration of hereditary angioedema (HAE) therapy, administered in Europe, Canada and the USA, were used to guide discussion at an international HAE expert meeting. The aim was to capture information about current practice in self-administered HAE therapy in these countries, including self-administration training, the key benefits of switching to self-administration, the barriers to self-administration and trends in self-administration. Overall, switching to self-administration therapy is looked upon favourably from both patient and clinician perspectives by virtue of the potential improvement in quality of life arising from optimisation of therapy and early intervention. The recent changes to product licences allowing self-administration provide additional options for the management of HAE.

Introduction

Hereditary angioedema (HAE) is a rare autosomal dominant disorder with an estimated prevalence between 1:10,000 and 1:50,000 [1]. The rarity of the disease means there are often delays in the diagnosis and treatment of HAE [2, 3], an example is a recent Danish survey which found that the mean diagnostic delay was 16 years [4]. In addition, even with a family history of HAE, family screening is not always undertaken which may further delay diagnosis [5].

HAE types I and II, the two most common forms, involve the deficiency or decrease in function of C1 esterase inhibitor (C1-INH), leading to spontaneous attacks of angioedema at various body sites, including the skin and abdomen, resulting in a significant negative impact on health-related quality of life [6]. Laryngeal attacks are less common but can prove to be the most dangerous and even fatal because of the risk of asphyxiation. Normally, HAE symptoms increase over 24 h and then subside over 24–72 h [6]. Patients may experience prodromal symptoms such as unusual fatigue, a rash on the arms and legs

KARGER

E-Mail karger@karger.com
www.karger.com/iaa

1018–2438/13/1615–0010$38.00/0

Correspondence to: Dr. Teresa Caballero
Hospital La Paz Institute for Health Research, IdiPaz
Paseo de la Castellana 261
ES–28046 Madrid (Spain)
E-Mail mteresa.caballero@idipaz.es

Table 1. Summary of approved HAE treatments for self-administration[a] [11–13, 15, 22–25]

Drug	Country	Date	Indicated for
Berinert	23 EU countries	2011	Self-administration for acute attacks
	USA	2012	Self-administration for acute attacks
	23 EU countries	2013	Short-term prophylaxis, including self-administration
Cinryze	USA	2009	Self-administration for prophylaxis
	EU	2011	Acute attacks, routine prevention and short-term prophylaxis, including self-administration
Icatibant	EU	2011	Self-administration for acute attacks
	USA	2011	Self-administration for acute attacks

[a] Approvals in countries that participated in the survey. HAE = Hereditary angioedema.

and muscle aches. In a US survey developed by staff and patients at Penn State University, Hershey Medical Center, and sent to 158 HAE patients (46 returned completed surveys), a majority (87%) of HAE patients reported having a prodromal symptom prior to an attack [7]. The recognition of prodromal symptoms could provide an opportunity for early treatment and faster resolution of attack episodes [8].

Plasma-derived C1-INH (Berinert) has been the first-line therapy for HAE for several decades in Europe [9]. Another plasma-derived C1-INH (Cinryze) has recently been launched and both products, along with Cetor [10], are now nanofiltered C1-INH concentrates licensed for self-administration [10–13]. Currently, there are other therapies available for HAE attacks: a subcutaneous bradykinin receptor blocker [icatibant (Firazyr)] indicated for self-administration [14, 15], a subcutaneous kallikrein inhibitor [ecallantide (Kalbitor); not approved in Europe and not indicated for self-administration] [16, 17], and recombinant C1-INH (rC1-INH; Rhucin, Ruconest; not indicated for self-administration) [18]. Two of these products, rC1-INH and ecallantide, carry an anaphylactic risk, which limits their use for self-administration [17, 19]. Treatment regimens may involve short- or long-term prophylaxis as well as on-demand treatment for acute HAE attacks. The options for HAE management and available therapies have been reviewed recently [19]. Treatment of attacks has conventionally been administered in hospital or by healthcare providers; however, recent guidelines advise that all HAE patients should be considered for self-administration therapy [20, 21].

Recent licence changes to some HAE therapies have provided excellent opportunities for more patients to switch to self-administered therapy (table 1) [11–13, 15, 22–25]. Home-based self-administration of HAE therapy permits rapid treatment in the early stages of an HAE attack and has been shown to reduce the duration of such attacks [26]. Early administration of Berinert and Firazyr has been shown to reduce the duration of an acute attack [27, 28]. Short-term prophylaxis used prior to a procedure or an important event and long-term prophylaxis are both amenable to self-administration and have been reviewed recently [6, 29].

The purpose of this study was to report the results of a survey and follow-up on feedback from an international HAE expert meeting into current self-administration practices in Europe, Canada and the USA.

Methods

An online survey was prepared to collate current experience and trends in the uptake and training of C1-INH self-administration. The survey consisted of 16 questions examining: current practices in self-administration training and HAE therapy, benefits/concerns relating to self-administration and current trends in self-administration use. The questions were assessed by a mixture of multiple choices and written (free text) answers (table 2). The survey was sent to 21 HAE centres across Europe, Canada and the USA, to include those experts and centres invited to participate in the international HAE expert meeting.

For further details of current guidelines, practicalities of administration and perceived challenges please refer to the articles within this supplement by Cicardi et al. [30], Symons et al. [31] and Boysen et al. [32], respectively.

Results and Discussion

Ten centres across Europe (n = 8), Canada (n = 1) and the USA (n = 1) responded to the survey and were represented at the international HAE expert meeting.

Current Practices in Self-Administration Training and HAE Therapy (P1–P6)

All the centres who responded to the survey (n = 10) offered self-administration as a therapy option to their patients. The experience in offering self-administration training varied within and between countries, with Germany having a much longer experience than, for example, Italy, where this approach is still in the early stages of development. The majority of centres (n = 9) provid-

Int Arch Allergy Immunol 2013;161(suppl 1):10–16
DOI: 10.1159/000351233

Table 2. Questions and assessments employed in the questionnaire 'HAE Self-Administration Survey'

No.	Question	Assessed by	Answer range
Current practices in self-administration training and HAE therapy (P)			
P1	Do you currently offer your HAE patients the option of self-administration (or administration by other non-healthcare professionals, e.g. a family member outside of the physician office/hospital)?	Multiple choice	Yes/no
P2	Who trains your patients for self-administration?	Multiple choice	You/your staff/home nursing agency
P3	If you offer self-administered therapy to your patients is it with:	Multiple choice	Firazyr/Berinert/Cinryze
P4	Did the recent licence change for Berinert to include self-administration change your practice behaviour?	Multiple choice	Yes/no/unaware of licence change
P5	Did the recent licence change for Firazyr to include self-administration change your practice behaviour?	Multiple choice	Yes/no/unaware of licence change
P6	In your opinion what are the main (top 3) requirements for a patient to qualify for self-administration?	Written answer	
Benefits/concerns relating to self-administration (B)			
B1	What are the key benefits of switching from assisted infusion of Berinert to self-administered therapy from your perspective and from a patient perspective?	Written answer	
B2	Does your patient's quality of life improve with self-administration?	Multiple choice	Yes/no
B3	Do you think cost reduction occurs with self-administration?	Multiple choice	Yes/no
B4	What features of self-administered Berinert therapy may make a patient less likely to switch and, in your opinion, how could these clinical/psychosocial barriers be addressed?	Written answer	
B5	What are your concerns regarding self-administration?	Multiple choice	Infection/contamination/air emboli/other drugs/monitoring/poor venous access/no strong concerns
B6	What are the main (top 3) hurdles to enable/train patients to self-administer Berinert?	Written answer	
B7	What activities/resources would be most valuable to improve patient uptake of self-administered Berinert?	Written answer	
Trends in self-administration use (T)			
T1	Is the share of patients learning/practising self-administration…	Multiple choice	Increasing/decreasing/not changing
T2	What percentage of your patients self-administers their treatment?	Multiple choice	0/10/25/50/75/90/100
T3	Please provide a rough estimate of the percentage of your patients who self-administer using Firazyr, Berinert or Cinryze (% of total number of patients on respective therapy).	Written answer	

HAE = Hereditary angioedema.

ed training to patients by centre staff (either physicians or nurses) whilst the US centre utilised home care agencies.

There are a wide variety of experiences in the development and implementation of training programmes and these are summarised in table 3.

Of the three therapies indicated for self-administration, Firazyr, Berinert and Cinryze, the survey indicated that Firazyr or Berinert were the most popular therapies offered for self-administration (fig. 1). At the time of the survey, Cinryze was not available in some of the countries that took part in the survey. At some centres (n = 7) patients were only offered Firazyr or Berinert, while at another centre patients were able to choose between Firazyr, Berinert or Cinryze. At the remaining two centres choice was limited to either Firazyr only or Berinert only.

Survey respondents were divided equally as to whether the recent licence changes to Firazyr and Berinert regarding possibility for self-administration had influenced practice behaviour: yes (n = 5) and no (n = 5). Three of the responders who answered 'yes' commented that these changes had made it easier to offer self-administration to

Table 3. Status of self-administration training programmes

Country	Development and practice of self-administration training programmes
Canada	- Patients are taking 2–3 h to train. - Shortage of nurses to perform the training.
France	- Angioedema reference centre nurses ran training programme: 95% of patients already trained for self-administering Firazyr subcutaneously for on-demand treatment of acute attacks. - Started intravenous home therapy training with a few patients: angioedema nurses will improve their skills with the help of a German team to be able to train patients for intravenous self-administration.
Germany	- Post-training checks. - Training should include discussions of side effects and actions.
Italy	- Relatively new to home therapy training. Eleven patients have been successfully trained in Sicily with help from haemophilia staff. - Yet to determine strategy for refresher training.
Spain	- Nurse-led training programmes, supervised by physicians with some patients trained with help from haemophilia staff. Includes several sessions, post-training checks or refresher sessions. - The majority of patients are self-administering Firazyr for on-demand treatment of acute HAE attacks and a minority are administering Berinert, some of which are using off-label for long-term treatment.
UK	- Training supervised by immunology specialist nurses; variable number of training sessions depending on route of administration (often a single session for subcutaneous, more for intravenous) and patient competency and confidence. Refresher course at clinic review.
USA	- Home therapy companies/agencies provide training.

HAE = Hereditary angioedema.

their HAE patients and would lead to an increase in the number of self-administering patients.

Since the licence changes, it was commented that more patients have been trained to self-administer 'Firazyr for acute attacks as the subcutaneous technique is easy for the patient'. It was also suggested that the licence changes for Berinert would make it easier to offer self-administration for an intravenous drug and that it would increase the number of patients that are offered Berinert during acute attacks and for long-term prophylaxis.

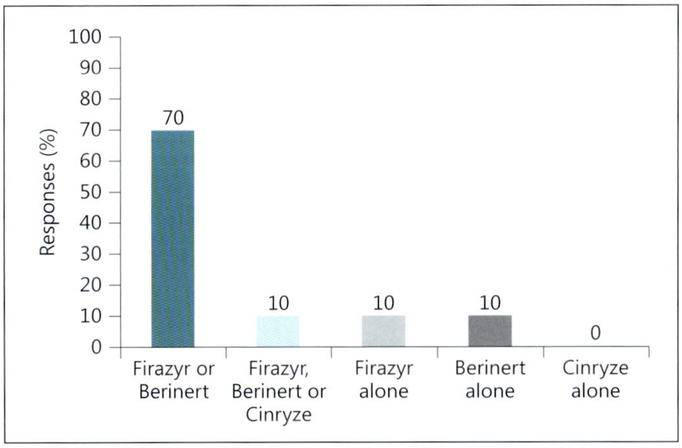

Fig. 1. Self-administration treatments offered by HAE clinical centres. At the time of the survey, Cinryze was not available in some of the countries surveyed.

The survey recorded 15 separate answers from respondents when asked what the three main requirements were for a patient to qualify for self-administration (fig. 2). The most popular answers were patient motivation, patient mental ability and clinical need. Notably, most of the requirements mentioned were patient related (60%) compared to clinical requirements (40%).

Key Benefits of Switching to Self-Administration (B1–B3)

The survey respondents agreed that self-administration improved patients' quality of life and outlined the key benefits as time saved, independence and convenience. From the clinicians' perspective the key benefits included early treatment, optimised therapy, lower dose and fewer visits to the emergency department. The benefits from the patients' perspective, as identified by the clinicians, included independence, convenience and more free time.

Cost savings were identified as a key benefit by all of the respondents, with savings in areas such as dose reduction due to early treatment, use of fewer resources at the physician's office and fewer visits to hospital emergency departments.

Barriers to Self-Administration (B4–B7)

Several barriers and concerns were perceived in relation to the introduction of self-administered HAE therapy, including funding and resource issues, legal/regulatory requirements and patient characteristics and functionality.

Legal and regulatory issues varied between countries and healthcare providers. For example, in Germany the

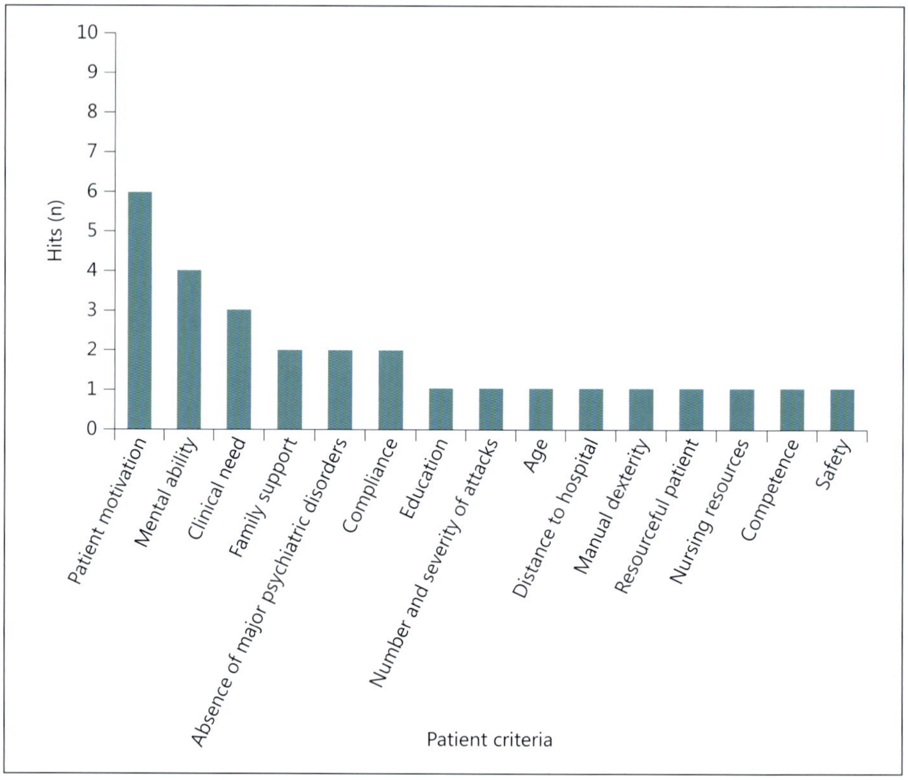

Fig. 2. Requirements for a patient to qualify for self-administration.

Table 4. Concerns regarding patient readiness to receive/switch to self-administration therapy

Concerns regarding patient ability to receive self-administration therapy
Mental ability
Inadequate education
Difficulty with administration
Age
Severe psychiatric disorders
Fear of self-injection
Distance to the hospital
Infrequent acute attacks
Willingness
Competency
No home care partner

prescribing physician remains legally responsible even though the treatment is being administered at home, either on-demand by the patient themselves or by a trained caregiver; this deters some physicians from prescribing self-administration therapy.

From the healthcare providers' perspective, barriers included: providing sufficient nurse resources, funding variations, keeping blood banks stocked with pasteurised-nanofiltered HAE products, the threat of increased infections and lack of therapy monitoring. Concerns were also raised about patients' readiness to switch to self-administration and the distance from home to their clinic (table 4). Patients who live close to the clinic would not see distance to the hospital as being a disadvantage; however, the benefits of self-administration in such situations would include a greater freedom to travel.

The physicians in the international HAE expert meeting commented that some of these issues can be addressed by providing sufficient training and support for self-administration, e.g. fears of intravenous or subcutaneous administration, difficulty in obtaining venous access and fear of self-injection.

Trends in Self-Administration (T1–T3)

All the centres reported that the number of patients learning/practising self-administration was increasing. No data were collected in relation to patients who, having tried self-administration, had reverted to hospital-based treatment or switched between different routes of administration i.e. intravenous or subcutaneous.

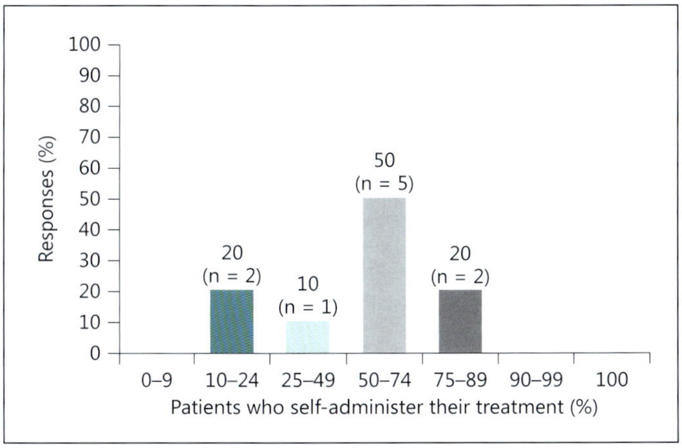

Fig. 3. Percentage of patients who are self-administering their treatment (across all centres).

The majority of centres (n = 7) reported that more than half (50–89%) of their patients were receiving self-administration therapy (fig. 3). As previously mentioned, most patients are offered a choice between Firazyr and Berinert, and these two products accounted for 96% of the HAE products used in self-administration (49% and 47%, respectively). Cinryze was reported to be used by a minority of patients (4%); however, at that time, Cinryze was not available in some of the countries that participated in the survey.

Conclusions

As the awareness of self-administration grows, an increasing number of patients are being offered and are using self-administration HAE therapy. Switching to self-administration therapy is looked upon favourably from both the patient [33] and clinician perspectives by virtue of the potential improvement in quality of life arising from optimisation of therapy and early intervention, with the total length of an attack being decreased with early intervention. However, future efforts should focus on encouraging more patients to take up self-administration and the key to this appears to be training in the skills needed, together with the availability of nurse/physician backup support, if required. Although some reference centres have initiated their own training programmes for patient self-administration, support should be provided, especially to centres dealing with small patient numbers.

A limitation of the survey was that it was restricted to those experts and centres invited to participate in the international HAE expert meeting, which could entail a selection bias. It should be noted that this survey largely reflects the current status of self-administration across Europe as 80% of the responding centres were European. Some centres also offered self-administration as an option to patients before it was licensed. Overall, in the majority of European countries, Berinert and Firazyr are equally used by patients opting for self-administration. However, national preferences may become apparent, for example in France where both Berinert and Firazyr are offered to patients, but most patients choose Firazyr for self-administration. The recent changes to product licences, which allow their use for self-administration, provide additional options for the management of HAE.

Disclosure Statement

Dr. Caballero has received speaker fees from Shire Human Genetic Therapies (HGT) Inc. and ViroPharma; consultancy fees from CSL Behring, Shire HGT Inc. and ViroPharma; funding for travel and meeting attendance from CSL Behring, Shire HGT Inc. and ViroPharma, and has participated in clinical trials for Dyax, Pharming, CSL Behring and Jerini AG/Shire HGT Inc.

Dr. Sala-Cunill speaks for Shire, consults for CSL Behring and Shire and does research for Shire, Pharming and ViroPharma.

Professor Cancian is a consultant for ViroPharma, Sobi, CSL Behring and Shire.

Dr. Craig speaks for CSL Behring, ViroPharma, Shire and Dyax. He does research for Pharming, CSL Behring, ViroPharma, Shire and Dyax. He is a consultant for CSL Behring and Dyax and has received educational grants from Dyax, ViroPharma and CSL Behring.

Prof. Neri has participated in advisory boards and symposia and has received educational grants from Shire, CSL Behring, ViroPharma and Pharming.

Dr. Keith has served on advisory boards for CSL Behring, Shire and ViroPharma. He has received research funding from Shire.

Dr. Boccon-Gibod has received consultancy fees from CSL Behring and Shire HGT Inc.

Dr. Bethune has been involved in advisory boards for Shire, ViroPharma and Swedish Orphan Biovitrum. She has received support to attend meetings from Shire, ViroPharma and CSL Behring. Her department has received support from Shire and CSL Behring.

Dr. Bork is a consultant for CSL Behring, Shire and ViroPharma.

References

1 Dagen C, Craig TJ: Treatment of hereditary angioedema: items that need to be addressed in practice parameter. Allergy Asthma Clin Immunol 2010;6:11.

2 Roche O, Blanch A, Caballero T, Sastre N, Callejo D, López-Trascasa M: Hereditary angioedema due to C1 inhibitor deficiency: patient registry and approach to the prevalence in Spain. Ann Allergy Asthma Immunol 2005;94:498–503.

3 Zuraw BL: Clinical practice. Hereditary angioedema. N Engl J Med 2008;359:1027–1036.
4 Bygum A: Hereditary angio-oedema in Denmark: a nationwide survey. Br J Dermatol 2009;161:1153–1158.
5 Lunn ML, Santos CB, Craig TJ: Is there a need for clinical guidelines in the United States for the diagnosis of hereditary angioedema and the screening of family members of affected patients? Ann Allergy Asthma Immunol 2010;104:211–214.
6 Cicardi M, Johnston DT: Hereditary and acquired complement component 1 esterase inhibitor deficiency: a review for the hematologist. Acta Haematol 2012;127:208–220.
7 Prematta MJ, Kemp JG, Gibbs JG, Mende C, Rhoads C, Craig TJ: Frequency, timing, and type of prodromal symptoms associated with hereditary angioedema attacks. Allergy Asthma Proc 2009;30:506–511.
8 Prematta MJ, Bewtra AK, Levy RJ, Wasserman RL, Jacobson KW, Machnig T, Craig TJ: Per-attack reporting of prodromal symptoms concurrent with C1-inhibitor treatment of hereditary angioedema attacks. Adv Ther 2012;29:913–922.
9 Bowen T, Cicardi M, Farkas H, Bork K, Longhurst HJ, Zuraw B, Aygoeren-Pürsün E, Craig T, Binkley K, Hebert J, Ritchie B, Bouillet L, Betschel S, Cogar D, Dean J, Devaraj R, Hamed A, Kamra P, Keith PK, Lacuesta G, Leith E, Lyons H, Mace S, Mako B, Neurath D, Poon MC, Rivard GE, Schellenberg R, Rowan D, Rowe A, Stark D, Sur S, Tsai E, Warrington R, Waserman S, Ameratunga R, Bernstein J, Björkander J, Brosz K, Brosz J, Bygum A, Caballero T, Frank M, Fust G, Harmat G, Kanani A, Kreuz W, Levi M, Li H, Martinez-Saguer I, Moldovan D, Nagy I, Nielsen EW, Nordenfelt P, Reshef A, Rusicke E, Smith-Foltz S, Späth P, Varga L, Xiang ZY: 2010 International consensus algorithm for the diagnosis, therapy and management of hereditary angioedema. Allergy Asthma Clin Immunol 2010;6:24.
10 HAEi: Sanquin Blood Supply Foundation has been granted marketing authorization for their plasma-derived C1-inhibitor product Cetor in Belgium, Luxembourg, France and Finland. 2010. http://www.haei.org/node/1181 (accessed 03 January 2013).
11 CSL Behring: CSL Behring receives European Health Authorities' approval for self-administration of Berinert®. 2011. http://www.cslbehring.com/news-room/european-health-authorities-approve-self-adminstration-of-berinert.htm (accessed 21 November 2012).
12 CSL Behring: CSL Behring receives FDA approval of expanded label on Berinert® for self-administration and treatment of acute laryngeal attacks of hereditary angioedema. 2012. http://www.cslbehring-us.com/news-room/HAE-Berinert-Self-Administration-and-Laryngeal-Attacks (accessed 21 November 2012).
13 ViroPharma Inc.: ViroPharma's Cinryze® (C1 inhibitor [human]) granted European marketing authorization for hereditary angioedema (HAE). 2011. http://ir.viropharma.com/releasedetail.cfm?ReleaseID=585060 (accessed 21 November 2012).
14 Cicardi M, Banerji A, Bracho F, Malbrán A, Rosenkranz B, Riedl M, Bork K, Lumry W, Aberer W, Bier H, Bas M, Greve J, Hoffmann TK, Farkas H, Reshef A, Ritchie B, Yang W, Grabbe J, Kivity S, Kreuz W, Levy RJ, Luger T, Obtulowicz K, Schmid-Grendelmeier P, Bull C, Sitkauskiene B, Smith WB, Toubi E, Werner S, Anné S, Björkander J, Bouillet L, Cillari E, Hurewitz D, Jacobson KW, Katelaris CH, Maurer M, Merk H, Bernstein JA, Feighery C, Floccard B, Gleich G, Hébert J, Kaatz M, Keith P, Kirkpatrick CH, Langton D, Martin L, Pichler C, Resnick D, Wombolt D, Fernández Romero DS, Zanichelli A, Arcoleo F, Knolle J, Kravec I, Dong L, Zimmermann J, Rosen K, Fan WT: Icatibant, a new bradykinin-receptor antagonist, in hereditary angioedema. N Engl J Med 2010;363:532–541.
15 Pharmiweb.com: European Commission approves self-administration label for Firazyr® (icatibant) for the symptomatic treatment of acute hereditary angioedema attacks. 2011. http://www.pharmiweb.com/PressReleases/pressrel.asp?ROW_ID=37878#axzz2Cm0UVl3D (accessed 21 November 2012).
16 Riedl M, Campion M, Horn PT, Pullman WE: Response time for ecallantide treatment of acute hereditary angioedema attacks. Ann Allergy Asthma Immunol 2010;105:430–436.
17 Caballero T, López-Serrano C: Anaphylactic reaction and antibodies to DX-88 (kallikrein inhibitor) in a patient with hereditary angioedema. J Allergy Clin Immunol 2006;117:476–477.
18 Zuraw B, Cicardi M, Levy RJ, Nuijens JH, Relan A, Visscher S, Haase G, Kaufman L, Hack CE: Recombinant human C1-inhibitor for the treatment of acute angioedema attacks in patients with hereditary angioedema. J Allergy Clin Immunol 2010;126:821–827.
19 Bork K: Current management options for hereditary angioedema. Curr Allergy Asthma Rep 2012;12:273–280.
20 Longhurst HJ, Farkas H, Craig T, Aygören-Pürsün E, Bethune C, Bjorkander J, Bork K, Bouillet L, Boysen H, Bygum A, Caballero T, Cicardi M, Dempster J, Gompels M, Gooi J, Grigoriadou S, Huffer U, Kreuz W, Levi MM, Long J, Martinez-Saguer I, Raguet M, Reshef A, Bowen T, Zuraw B: HAE international home therapy consensus document. Allergy Asthma Clin Immunol 2010;6:22.
21 Cicardi M, Bork K, Caballero T, Craig T, Li HH, Longhurst H, Reshef A, Zuraw B, HAWK: Evidence-based recommendations for the therapeutic management of angioedema owing to hereditary C1 inhibitor deficiency: consensus report of an International Working Group. Allergy 2012;67:147–157.
22 Food and Drug Administration: FDA approves Firazyr to treat acute attacks of hereditary angioedema. 2011. http://www.fda.gov/newsevents/newsroom/pressannouncements/ucm269616.htm (accessed 20 September 2012).
23 CSL Behring: CSL Behring received MHRA approval for self-administration of Berinert® (C1 esterase inhibitor, human). 2012. http://www.cslbehring.co.uk/s1/cs/beuk/1161072713064/news/1255928888774/prdetail.htm (accessed 21 November 2012).
24 CSL Behring: CSL Behring receives European Health Authorities' approval of Berinert® for short-term prophylaxis in adults and children. 2013. http://www.cslbehring.com/s1/cs/enco/1151517263302/news/1255931201677/prdetail.htm (accessed 17 April 2013).
25 ViroPharma Inc.: ViroPharma receives Complete Response letter for Cinryze™ supplemental Biologics License Application for acute treatment of hereditary angioedema. 2009. http://ir.viropharma.com/releasedetail.cfm?ReleaseID=543136 (accessed 21 November 2012).
26 Levi M, Choi G, Picavet C, Hack CE: Self-administration of C1-inhibitor concentrate in patients with hereditary or acquired angioedema caused by C1-inhibitor deficiency. J Allergy Clin Immunol 2006;117:904–908.
27 Bork K, Staubach P, Bernstein JA, Feuersenger H, Machnig T, Craig TJ: Efficacy of C1-inhibitor concentrate (Berinert®) for the treatment of cutaneous attacks of acute hereditary angioedema compared to historical untreated controls. J Allergy Clin Immunol 2013;131:AB31.
28 Maurer M, Aberer W, Bouillet L, Caballero T, Fabien V, Kanny G, Kaplan A, Longhurst H, Zanichelli A, IOS Investigators: Hereditary angioedema attacks resolve faster and are shorter after early icatibant treatment. PLoS ONE 2013;8:e53773.
29 Costantino G, Casazza G, Bossi I, Duca P, Cicardi M: Long-term prophylaxis in hereditary angio-oedema: a systematic review. BMJ Open 2012;2:e000524.
30 Cicardi M, Craig T, Martinez-Saguer I, Hébert J, Longhurst HJ: Review of recent guidelines and consensus statements on hereditary angioedema therapy with focus on self-administration. Int Arch Allergy Immunol 2013;161(suppl 1):3–9.
31 Symons C, Rossi O, Magerl M, Andritschke K: Practical approac to self-administration of intravenous C1-INH concentrate: a nursing perspective. Int Arch Allergy Immunol 2013;161(suppl 1):17–20.
32 Boysen HB, Bouillet L, Aygören-Pürsün E: Challenges of C1-inhibitor concentrate self-administration. Int Arch Allergy Immunol 2013;161(suppl 1):21–25.
33 Boccon-Gibod I, Bouillet L: Safety and efficacy of icatibant self-administration for acute hereditary angioedema. Clin Exp Immunol 2012;168:303–307.

Original Paper

International Archives of Allergy and Immunology

Int Arch Allergy Immunol 2013;161(suppl 1):17–20
DOI: 10.1159/000351236

Published online: May 28, 2013

Practical Approach to Self-Administration of Intravenous C1-INH Concentrate: A Nursing Perspective

C. Symons[a] O. Rossi[b] M. Magerl[c] K. Andritschke[d]

[a]Derriford Hospital, Plymouth, UK; [b]University of Florence, Florence, Italy; [c]Department of Dermatology and Allergy, Charité – Universitätsmedizin, Berlin, and [d]Haemophilia Centre Rhein Main, Mörfelden, Germany

Key Words

Hereditary angioedema · Self-administration · Practicalities

Abstract

At an international hereditary angioedema (HAE) expert meeting, results from a survey were used to guide discussion on how best to advise patients on self-administering intravenous C1 esterase inhibitor therapy. Treatment differences across Europe were highlighted, together with the practicalities of self-administration and useful resources for patients in the future. The international HAE experts noted an increase in the uptake of self-administration, with patients being trained by nursing staff. All patients who are willing and able to self-administer should be offered this treatment option and patients should be encouraged to treat attacks early. Several initiatives were suggested regarding support for patients who self-administer therapy, including a 24-hour helpline and home care agencies.

Introduction

Until recently, it was common practice in most countries that hereditary angioedema (HAE) patients had to present at hospital for the treatment of an attack. However, treatment options for the management of HAE have advanced, with products now licensed for self-administration being offered to patients, for example. Here we discuss practical approaches to self-administration of intravenous C1 esterase inhibitor (C1-INH), with advice gained by consensus at an international HAE expert meeting held in June 2012.

Methods

To assess the current practice of HAE self-administration treatment across Europe, a survey was sent to a group of experts in the field of HAE (including physicians, nurses and a patient-expert) prior to attendance at an international HAE expert meeting, organised for the purpose of seeking advice on current practice in self-administration treatment of HAE. For further details of the survey, refer to the supplement article by Caballero et al. [1] entitled 'Current status of implementation of self-administration training programmes in various regions of Europe, Canada and the USA in the management of hereditary angioedema'. At the international HAE expert meeting the results of the questionnaire were used to direct discussion. Participants considered how best to advise patients on self-administering intravenous C1-INH treatment.

Treatment Differences across Europe

Consensus documents recommend administration of pasteurised-nanofiltered C1-INH for short- (STP) and long-term prophylaxis (LTP) and pasteurised-nanofil-

Correspondence to: Sr. Christine Symons
Derriford Hospital, Plymouth Hospitals NHS Trust
Derriford Road
Plymouth PL6 8DH (UK)
E-Mail Christine.symons1@nhs.net

Table 1. Guidelines versus current practice

Guidelines	Current practice
– For acute attacks, every patient with HAE should have the immediate means to control the attack. – Several products have been licensed for self-administration therapy including pasteurised-nanofiltered C1-INH (Berinert and Cinryze) and Firazyr. Kalbitor can be administered in the home by a healthcare provider. – Observational studies demonstrate faster relief and reduced attack severity when C1-INH is given early.	– Pasteurised-nanofiltered C1-INH and Firazyr were identified from the survey as being the most regularly used for administration.
– For STP, guidelines recommend the administration of pasteurised-nanofiltered C1-INH before any major procedures or intubation and it should be immediately available for minor manipulations. If C1-INH is not available, attenuated androgens should be used.	– International HAE expert meeting discussion identified that, for STP with androgens, all physicians were treating 5–7 days prior to any procedure and 2–5 days after a procedure.
– For LTP, pasteurised-nanofiltered C1-INH concentrate is detailed as the safest long-term approach. It is feasible to use attenuated androgens such as danazol or stanozolol; however, they are associated with several side effects.	– For LTP, participants were commonly using pasteurised-nanofiltered C1-INH; however, androgens were often used, possibly due to their availability, but were associated with severe side effects, most notably in women. – For prophylaxis, European participants are using androgens or tranexamic acid (due to minimal side effects, availability and cost).

C1-INH = C1 esterase inhibitor; HAE = hereditary angioedema; LTP = long-term prophylaxis; STP = short-term prophylaxis.

tered C1-INH, icatibant (Firazyr) and ecallantide (Kalbitor) for acute attacks [2]; however, current practice indicates that other products are regularly being used (table 1).

Currently in Spain, France and Germany pasteurised-nanofiltered C1-INH is only approved for use when oral treatment for prophylaxis has failed or on-demand use does not control a patient sufficiently. It was also commented that patient consent is needed in Spain for LTP. In the UK, Italy and Canada, consent is needed to prescribe and document the use of blood products. Although participants used a variety of products, the consensus concluded that the goal of treatment was to treat patients early in an attack. Another factor is cost and reimbursement. In the USA, hospitals charge more for use of a therapy than it costs to purchase but some care packages do not allow self-administration therapy. The economic burden associated with HAE has a significant effect on patients, healthcare systems and society [3]. Analysis of costs by Wilson et al. [4] indicated the largest component of direct cost is hospital stays followed by emergency department visits for acute attacks, whereas the main component of indirect costs varies with attack severity [4].

Administration

The international HAE expert panel identified self-administration as a means to intervene early in acute attacks and give patients control of their own treatment. It was highlighted by the patient-expert that patients prefer the term self-administration over the term home therapy as it removes the connotation of being restricted to the home for administration.

Due to limited experience in Europe, patients are often treated in haemophilia and immunology/allergy centres, where the nursing staff teach administration techniques to HAE healthcare providers. In the UK, there is a wide experience of treating and training patients for self-administration both with hospital staff and home care nurses. In the USA, home care agencies are used to train patients and can follow-up with them in their homes. Participants from centres in Canada and Germany discussed the difficulties with smaller clinics and the need for nurse training programmes.

As noted in guidelines by Longhurst et al. [2], training should be conducted over several sessions to ensure the patient, and any treatment partner, have had sufficient practice to be familiar and confident with the technical and medical aspects of self-administration [2]. In practice, a variety of training sessions were offered (table 2).

Overall, the speed at which patients were learning the necessary skill set was surprising, often only taking a few hours. For follow-up training sessions, legislation varies between countries, with some permitting hospital staff access to patients' homes, such as in the UK and Germany, or facilitated by home care agencies in the USA. To improve follow-up in Europe, it was recommended that the use of home care agencies or the addition of a home care option for hospital staff may be worth investing in to help improve patient management. Clinicians were reassured that once the skills have been acquired by a patient they are retained long-term and that frequency of administration alone is not in itself a reason to disregard a self-treatment option.

Practicalities of Administration

Although consensus documents recommend early treatment of attacks at all sites, this is not thought to be practised (table 3). Patients need to be encouraged not to endure attacks even if they believe they can cope, but to treat them early.

All patients who are willing and capable to do so should be offered self-administration therapy; the skill to self-administer can be life-saving. The questionnaire circulated prior to the international HAE expert meeting identified that between 50–74% of physicians' patients are self-administering and that the nursing staff are the main points of contact for training.

International HAE expert consensus agreed that for training purposes, patients are allowed to have with them a 'buddy' who will be able to help with self-administration if required. Initially, patients are taught how to reconstitute the lyophilised product and are talked through the process of intravenous administration and the equipment they need. Patients are then shown how to prepare the equipment and the infusion site, and are shown the technique to infuse. Most patients choose to inject intravenously into their forearm; however, this can sometimes be difficult if the patient is in pain or has hand or eye swelling, which is why the 'trained buddy' may be helpful. To minimise vessel damage, a 25-gauge butterfly needle is recommended for administration. Patients are also advised that they should keep their preferred vein for self-infusion and they should avoid allowing others to administer intravenous drugs or blood products into their preferred vein.

To aid patients with administration, pharmaceutical companies provide kits that contain a set of components

Table 2. Training regimens

Country	Training regimen
Canada	– Patients are taking approximately 2–3 h to train. – Shortage of nurses for training.
Germany	Several programmes were identified, range includes: – 3–4 h to become proficient (e.g. 2 h on first visit and 1–1.5 h on second visit). – 3 to 4 sessions with up to 2 h per session to train patients.
Italy	– Relatively new to self-administration therapy. – Training programmes managed by physicians and nurses.
Spain	– Relatively new to self-administration therapy. – Training programmes initiated with help from haemophilia staff. – Some centres offer up to 7 training sessions.
UK	– Single training session offered followed by a refresher course.
USA	– Home care agencies provide training.

Table 3. Attack treatment sites

Country	Attack site treated
Canada	– Abdominal and laryngeal attacks are always treated. – Peripheral attacks are treated depending on severity and frequency; this decision is left to the patient.
Germany	– Patients experiencing wandering attacks (i.e. an attack that starts in the arm and moves to the face) are encouraged to treat as an attack that can spread anywhere.
Italy	– Patients experiencing wandering attacks (i.e. an attack that starts in the arm and moves to the face) are encouraged to treat as an attack that can spread anywhere.
Spain	– Attacks are treated depending on the severity; mild attacks go untreated. – Recently, more peripheral attacks are being treated. Patients can decide if they want to treat.
UK	– Patients do not always treat themselves for mild attacks. – Participants agreed they need to break the culture of not treating as they are used to it (able to cope) and that they should encourage patients to treat all attacks (as any attack can become severe).
USA	– Some patients do not treat mild attacks, but the consensus suggests they should.

Int Arch Allergy Immunol 2013;161(suppl 1):17–20
DOI: 10.1159/000351236

for dosing. Not all countries require all components because some are supplied in the clinic. Based on feedback from patients, some changes could be made to improve convenience. For example, tubing length could be made longer to aid infusion, or syringes with a larger volume could be used to avoid syringe change; changing the syringe can be challenging for the patient. Patients find the Mix2Vials (Medimop Medical Projects) a very easy system to use, although they are not available in all countries. Other key issues relating to self-administration are discussed in this supplement by Boysen et al. [5] ('Challenges of C1-INH concentrate self-administration').

Intravenous routes of self-administration do not appear to pose a problem for the majority of patients. The international HAE expert meeting members commented that patients like to have the flexibility of intravenous and subcutaneous administration routes as they can select the method appropriate for their setting. For example, people who are travelling find that subcutaneous self-administration is more discreet.

For treatment of children, the participating physicians felt that it was good practice to teach children when they are young as it can help in overcoming any fear of self-administration. Siblings of the child can assist with teaching them how to self-administer and act as a 'buddy'. In Europe, pasteurised-nanofiltered C1-INH is considered to be a treatment of choice for acute attacks in paediatric patients with HAE as well as for STP and LTP [2, 6].

Patient Resources

In identifying requirements for further training resources, the use of haemophilia and immunoglobulin centres to aid nurse and patient training was recommended. As patients may not have regular contact with a nurse, a 24-hour helpline (as available in haemophilia centres) was also suggested. As patients may forget parts of their training when they are on their own, a check sheet may help to ensure all kit is prepared appropriately and all steps followed in the correct sequence.

Conclusion

The international HAE experts noted an increased uptake of self-administration, with patients being trained by nursing staff. Nurses have an important role in the training and guidance of patients and as more patients take up self-administration, experience will continue to grow. Where there is minimal experience to date, nurses and patients are attending haemophilia and immunology clinics to learn administration techniques. The experience of haemophilia and immunology nurses needs to be shared across departments, especially within smaller clinics. As patients may not be trained by their regular nurse, a 24-hour helpline may be a useful additional resource for patients. So as patients do not feel tied to the home, the term self-administration is preferred over home therapy and we encourage people to use this term when appropriate.

Disclosure Statement

Sr. Symons has been supported by Shire, ViroPharma and CSL Behring.

Dr. Rossi has received funding from CSL Behring to attend meetings.

Dr. Magerl is, or recently was, a speaker and/or advisor for CSL Behring, Shire/Jerini, Pharming, ViroPharma, Swedish Orphan Biovitrum, Faes Pharma, Uriach and Moxy GmbH.

Ms. Andritschke has participated in advisory boards for CSL Behring.

References

1 Caballero T, Sala-Cunill A, Cancian M, Craig TJ, Neri S, Keith PK, Boccon-Gibod I, Bethune C, Bork K: Current status of implementation of self-administration training in various regions of Europe, Canada and the USA in the management of hereditary angioedema. Int Arch Allergy Immunol 2013;161(suppl 1):10–16.

2 Longhurst HJ, Farkas H, Craig T, Aygören-Pürsün E, Bethune C, Bjorkander J, Bork K, Bouillet L, Boysen H, Bygum A, Caballero T, Cicardi M, Dempster J, Gompels M, Gooi J, Grigoriadou S, Huffer U, Kreuz W, Levi MM, Long J, Martinez-Saguer I, Raguet M, Reshef A, Bowen T, Zuraw B: HAE international home therapy consensus document. Allergy Asthma Clin Immunol 2010;6:22.

3 HAEi International Patient Organization for C1 Inhibitor Deficiencies: State of management of HAE in Europe. 2011. http://www.haeday.org/sites/default/files/upload/English%20PDF-%20HAEi_Report.pdf (accessed 24 September 2012).

4 Wilson DA, Bork K, Shea EP, Rentz AM, Blaustein MB, Pullman WE: Economic costs associated with acute attacks and long-term management of hereditary angioedema. Ann Allergy Asthma Immunol 2010;104:314–320.

5 Boysen HB, Bouillet L, Aygören-Pürsün E: Challenges of C1-inhibitor concentrate self-administration. Int Arch Allergy Immunol 2013;161(suppl 1):21–25.

6 Wahn V, Aberer W, Eberl W, Fasshauer M, Kühne T, Kurnik K, Magerl M, Meyer-Olson D, Martinez-Saguer I, Späth P, Staubach-Renz P, Kreuz W: Hereditary angioedema (HAE) in children and adolescents – a consensus on therapeutic strategies. Eur J Pediatr 2012;171:1339–1348.

Original Paper

International Archives of Allergy and Immunology

Int Arch Allergy Immunol 2013;161(suppl 1):21–25
DOI: 10.1159/000351238

Published online: May 28, 2013

Challenges of C1-Inhibitor Concentrate Self-Administration

H.B. Boysen[a] L. Bouillet[b] E. Aygören-Pürsün[c]

[a]Executive Director of HAEi, Aarhus, Denmark; [b]National Reference Center of Angioedema, Grenoble University Hospital, Grenoble, France; [c]Johann Wolfgang Goethe-University Hospital, Frankfurt, Germany

Key Words

Hereditary angioedema · Self-administration · Barriers · Challenges · Quality of life

Abstract

Self-administration of therapy can help hereditary angioedema (HAE) patients regain control of their disease or reduce its impact and improve the quality of their lives. However, data from a self-administration survey, and subsequent discussion at an international HAE expert meeting, identified several barriers to self-administration therapy. These barriers include difficulty in administration technique, availability of nursing resources and the mental capacity of the patient. Encouragingly, international HAE experts identified that once a patient has acquired self-administration skills, they generally retain them in the long-term. As patient uptake increases, it was recommended that follow-up management plans should be established to address any issues from the patient's perspective.

Introduction

Awareness of hereditary angioedema (HAE) is extremely low and diagnosis of the condition may take several years with a mean delay to diagnosis of as much as 16 years [1]. This emphasises the urgent need to raise awareness of the disease among clinicians and within families who carry a hereditary predisposition to the condition. Surprisingly, family screening is not always performed despite HAE being an autosomal dominant disease with 50% penetrance [2].

The mechanisms underlying an HAE attack remain relatively unknown and the severity of symptoms is highly variable both within and between patients. Episodes of swelling can occur in the extremities, face, trunk, airways or abdominal areas (fig. 1). The uncertainty of timing, severity and length of an HAE attack can cause great anxiety for patients given that the swelling can be fatal if it occurs in the larynx; the risk of dying from an airway obstruction, if left untreated, has been estimated to approach 40% [3].

Currently, the management of HAE focuses on providing rapid relief or prevention of symptoms during an attack. Treatment options approved in Europe for acute attacks include plasma-derived C1 esterase inhibitor (C1-INH) concentrate (Berinert, Cetor and Cinryze), recombinant C1-INH (Rhucin, Ruconest) and bradykinin β_2 receptor antagonist [icatibant (Firazyr)]. Long-term prophylaxis is approved with C1-INH concentrate (Cinryze) and also traditionally involves antifibrinolytics or androgens (e.g. danazol or stanozolol), although approval varies across Europe. Until recently, patients had to visit the clinic, emergency department or hospital for treatment. The option of self-administration is now being offered to patients as it is thought that this therapy option can help

Correspondence to: Mr. Henrik Boysen
International Patient Organization for C1 Inhibitor Deficiencies
Soenderholmvej 158, Bering
DK–8361 Hasselager (Denmark)
E-Mail h.boysen@haei.org

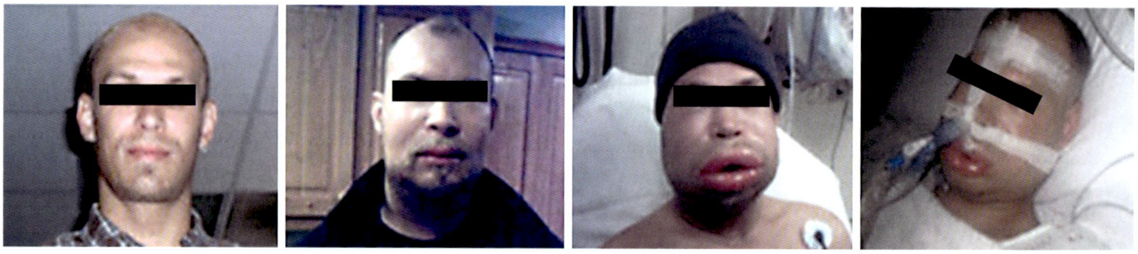

Fig. 1. Progression of an HAE attack (image source, Bygum et al. [1]).

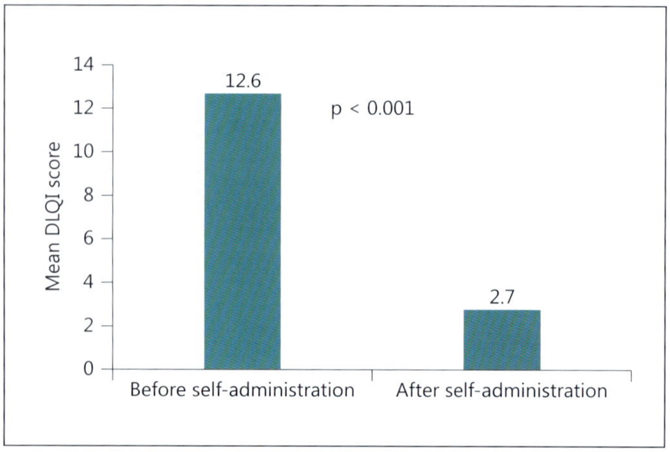

Fig. 2. Mean DLQI score of 7 patients before and after self-administration HAE therapy [6]. DLQI = Dermatology life quality index.

patients regain control/reduce the impact of disease and improve the quality of their lives [4].

Several studies have explored the impact of HAE on health-related quality of life. Some investigations used the short form 36 (SF-36) and also the dermatology life quality index (DLQI), which are useful for comparing HAE to other diseases [5, 6]. Investigations show that self-administration of treatment was associated with improvements in the mean DLQI score ($p < 0.001$; fig. 2) and in both physical ($p = 0.0001$) and psychological parameters ($p = 0.0033$) on the SF-36 [6]. More recently, disease-specific questionnaires have been developed [7, 8] which aim to specifically assess health-related quality of life in HAE patients.

Methods

To assess the current practice of HAE self-administration treatment across Europe, Canada and the USA, a survey was sent to a group of experts in the field of HAE (including physicians, nurses and a patient-expert) prior to attendance at an international HAE expert meeting organised for the purpose of seeking advice on current practice in self-administration treatment of HAE. For further details of the survey refer to the paper by Caballero et al. [9] in this supplement ('Current status of implementation of self-administration training programmes in various regions of Europe, Canada and the USA in the management of hereditary angioedema'). At the international HAE expert meeting the results of the questionnaire were used to direct discussion. In particular, participants considered some of the challenges that physicians, nurses and patients face and how they may be overcome.

Challenges and Solutions

International HAE expert meeting participants believed all HAE patients should be considered for self-administration if the patient is willing; however, some patients may need more support than others and some may not be eligible for self-administration. The main challenge identified for self-administration patients was obtaining the necessary skill set (fig. 3). Discussion identified that once a patient has acquired the skills for administration, for both intravenous and subcutaneous infusion, they generally retain them as a long-term competency. The time between attacks is not a reason to not offer a patient the option to self-administer.

The current guidelines for treatment indicate that all patients should participate in a training programme over several sessions to ensure that patients and, if applicable, a training partner, have had sufficient practice to be familiar and confident with the technical and medical aspects of self-administration [10]. The clinical experts revealed that patients were learning the necessary skill set faster than expected and that it was common practice that patients attended a training session for 2 h followed by a follow-up session, as described elsewhere in this supplement (see Symons et al. [11] 'Practical approach to self-administration of intravenous C1-INH

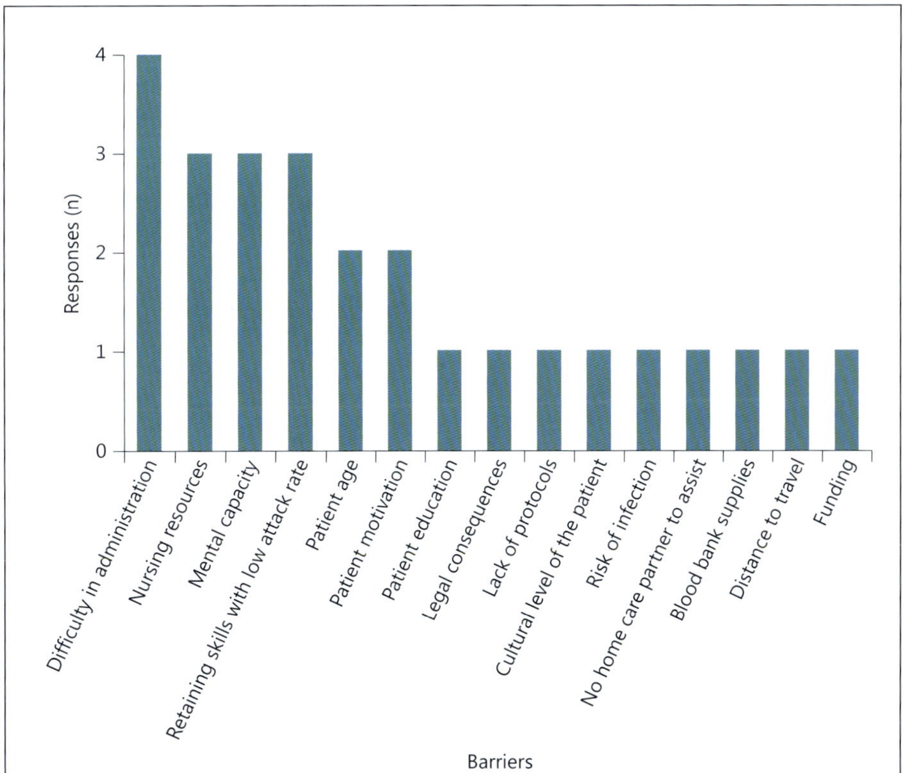

Fig. 3. What are the main hurdles to enable/train patients to self-administer Berinert?

concentrate: a nursing perspective' for details of training schedules).

For self-administration, patients are responsible for self-diagnosis of an attack and, although rare, there is the risk of misinterpretation. Patients are thought to be aware of the onset of an attack, allowing ample time to administer therapy and minimise the severity and length of an attack. Clinical experts at the international HAE expert meeting recommended reporting all attacks and any unusual or lingering symptoms to ensure there are no untreated symptoms. Monitoring of attacks may also help assess a patient's ability to manage their disease state. The decreased contact between patient and physician is addressed by having agreed follow-up visits to assess progress and to review the patient reports. International HAE expert meeting participants discussed the timing between patient visits; initially once every 3 months was recommended to ensure correct management of their condition, followed by once every 6 months when the patient was more comfortable with self-administration. For the benefit of patient and physician, it was agreed that an acute action plan should be arranged to permit the patient to take appropriate action if self-administration is ineffective.

Due to the rarity and potential severity of the disease, more needs to be done to raise awareness of the condition amongst physicians. At the international HAE expert meeting, it was remarked that some patients reported not attending hospital during an attack because the time to treatment could be delayed by a lack of HAE experience of the treating physician in the emergency department. It was reported that many physicians do not understand the disease and they would often administer therapy directed at histamine-induced angioedema instead of the appropriate therapy. Indeed, some physicians do not understand the urgency for treatment if the attack is not likely to be fatal. In discussion, the need for acute action treatment plans for the patient and the treating physician were stressed. In raising awareness of the condition, patients may get the rapid response they need, which could potentially be life-saving.

Increasing awareness of HAE may also lead to better facilities being provided for patients who have to learn how to self-administer treatment. Advice from the participants was that there are only a minority of places with good facilities. This makes self-infusion a challenge for new patients to learn. In addition, because not all attacks occur in the home, it is often difficult to self-administer

Int Arch Allergy Immunol 2013;161(suppl 1):21–25
DOI: 10.1159/000351238

Table 1. Guidance on HAE self-administration therapy

Key information	Reasons for usefulness
Administer treatment prior to an attack	This will help to prevent an attack or lead to rapid recovery and minimal attack duration.
Administer treatment early and when hydrated	This will aid infusion to ensure full treatment is achieved rapidly.
Avoid central lines	Infection rates are generally very low but increase with the use of central lines; avoid them to minimise infection rates.

HAE = Hereditary angioedema.

Table 2. Advantages and disadvantages of prescribing self-administration HAE therapy

Advantages	Disadvantages
Able to treat an attack rapidly which minimises days off work or school	Decreased patient/physician contact
Able to manage own disease	Fear of self-infusion
Able to travel	Training session required
Improved patient quality of life	May find it difficult to obtain venous access
Subcutaneous infusion is more discreet than intravenous infusion	

HAE = Hereditary angioedema.

medication with some patients choosing not to infuse as they do not want to be seen injecting in public.

The final barrier discussed at the international HAE expert meeting was the legal ramifications of offering self-infusion to patients in some European countries. For example, in Germany, the prescribing physician is responsible for the patient regardless of the location of treatment and therefore not all physicians will encourage self-administration. More needs to be done to demonstrate that self-administration is a viable option and that self-diagnosis and self-administration may be beneficial to the patient by reducing the time to treatment, decreasing attack severity and improving time to recovery. The convenience of self-administration and the independence that stems from this also improves patients' quality of life. In accordance with the current guidelines, all voluntary patients should be considered for self-administration and, after discussion, a decision should be made if the patient is willing and able to self-administer therapy [10]. Discussion of treatment management with patients during regular check-ups should allow patients and physicians to come to a mutual agreement that suits both parties.

Factors to Help Those Newly Diagnosed with HAE

Treatment of an HAE attack can be a daunting process. Discussion at the international HAE expert meeting highlighted a number of key points to aid self-administration, as shown in table 1.

Self-administration enables patients to have control of their disease management. Patients feel in control of their lives with self-treatment enabling them to lead a normal life, being able to work and travel and minimising days off from work or school.

As with all treatments there are advantages and disadvantages; however, the advantages outweigh the disadvantages (table 2). The options for self-administration treatment include intravenous and subcutaneous infusion which enables patients to select the most appropriate one for their needs. Many patients find the independence and improved quality of life gained with self-infusion empowers them to manage the disease instead of being managed by it.

Conclusion

Raising the awareness of HAE amongst healthcare providers globally may help increase diagnosis and treatment of HAE. With the increase in treatment options and approvals for self-administration, physicians are beginning to offer self-administration as a viable treatment option that should be considered for all HAE patients. As patient uptake increases, a follow-up management plan should be established to address any issues from the patient's perspective and to identify key areas for follow-up. Having the choice of when and where to self-administer provides the flexibility needed for successful treatment. Experience with self-administration to date suggests that patients should have the confidence that most challenges they encounter can be resolved by their educated local nurse or treating physician.

Disclosure Statement

Mr. Boysen is the Executive Director of HAEi – International Patient Organization for C1 Inhibitor Deficiencies, which has received or receives unrestricted educational funding from CMIC Holdings Co., CSL Behring, Dyax Corp., Santarus Inc., Shire, Sigma-Tau Group, Sobi – Swedish Orphan Biovitrum and ViroPharma Incorporated.

Dr. Bouillet has received honorarium from CSL Behring, Shire and ViroPharma for attending advisory boards and conferences.

Dr. Aygören-Pürsün has been involved in consultancy work and advisory boards for CSL Behring, Shire, ViroPharma and Sobi and has received grants and given lectures/spoken at symposia for CSL Behring, Shire and ViroPharma.

References

1 Bygum A, Aygören-Pürsün E, Caballero T, Beusterien K, Gholizadeh S, Musingarimi P, Wait S, Boysen H: The hereditary angioedema burden of illness study in Europe (HAE-BOIS-Europe): background and methodology. BMC Dermatol 2012;12:4.

2 Lunn ML, Santos CB, Craig TJ: Is there a need for clinical guidelines in the United States for the diagnosis of hereditary angioedema and the screening of family members of affected patients? Ann Allergy Asthma Immunol 2010;104:211–214.

3 Bork K, Siedlecki K, Bosch S, Schopf RE, Kreuz W: Asphyxiation by laryngeal edema in patients with hereditary angioedema. Mayo Clin Proc 2000;75:349–354.

4 HAEi International Patient Organization for C1 Inhibitor Deficiencies: State of management of HAE in Europe. 2011. http://www.haeday.org/sites/default/files/upload/English%20PDF-%20HAEi_Report.pdf (accessed 24 September 2012).

5 Lumry WR, Castaldo AJ, Vernon MK, Blaustein MB, Wilson DA, Horn PT: The humanistic burden of hereditary angioedema: Impact on health-related quality of life, productivity, and depression. Allergy Asthma Proc 2010;31:407–414.

6 Bygum A, Andersen KE, Mikkelsen CS: Self-administration of intravenous C1-inhibitor therapy for hereditary angioedema and associated quality of life benefits. Eur J Dermatol 2009;19:147–151.

7 Prior N, Remor E, Gómez-Traseira C, López-Serrano C, Cabañas R, Contreras J, Campos Á, Cardona V, Cimbollek S, González-Quevedo T, Guilarte M, de Rojas DH, Marcos C, Rubio M, Tejedor-Alonso MÁ, Caballero T: Development of a disease-specific quality of life questionnaire for adult patients with hereditary angioedema due to C1 inhibitor deficiency (HAE-QoL): Spanish multi-centre research project. Health Qual Life Outcomes 2012;10:82.

8 Weller K, Groffik A, Magerl M, Tohme N, Martus P, Krause K, Metz M, Staubach P, Maurer M: Development and construct validation of the angioedema quality of life questionnaire. Allergy 2012;67:1289–1298.

9 Caballero T, Sala-Cunill A, Cancian M, Craig TJ, Neri S, Keith PK, Boccon-Gibod I, Bethune C, Bork K: Current status of implementation of self-administration training in various regions of Europe, Canada and the USA in the management of HAE. Int Arch Allergy Immunol 2013;161(suppl 1):10–16.

10 Longhurst HJ, Farkas H, Craig T, Aygören-Pürsün E, Bethune C, Bjorkander J, Bork K, Bouillet L, Boysen H, Bygum A, Caballero T, Cicardi M, Dempster J, Gompels M, Gooi J, Grigoriadou S, Huffer U, Kreuz W, Levi MM, Long J, Martinez-Saguer I, Raguet M, Reshef A, Bowen T, Zuraw B: HAE international home therapy consensus document. Allergy Asthma Clin Immunol 2010;6:22.

11 Symons C, Rossi O, Magerl M, Andritschke K: Practical approach to self-administration of intravenous C1-INH concentrate: a nursing perspective. Int Arch Allergy Immunol 2013;161(suppl 1):17–20.

International Archives of
Allergy and Immunology

Int Arch Allergy Immunol 2013;161(suppl 1):26–27
DOI: 10.1159/000351241

Published online: May 28, 2013

Recent Advances in Hereditary Angioedema Self-Administration Treatment: Summary of an International Hereditary Angioedema Expert Meeting

Timothy J. Craig

College of Medicine, Penn State University, Hershey Medical Center, Hershey, Pa., USA

A significant amount of progress has been made in recent years in the understanding and treatment of hereditary angioedema (HAE), with more products being licensed for use worldwide (table 1). With the recent registration and introduction of pasteurised-nanofiltered C1 esterase inhibitor for self-administration, patients have new treatment opportunities and an increasing number of healthcare providers are offering more patients the option of self-administration therapy. However, the international HAE expert meeting demonstrated slow uptake of this treatment option. In general, we need to increase awareness of the benefits of self-administration and encourage patients to enter training programmes linked to self-injection of treatment.

As discussed in the article by Cicardi et al. [1], the guidelines for HAE diagnosis and treatment have progressed over the years, with recent guidelines often reflecting current practice in the majority of areas, including for self-administration. As identified through both the guidelines and the international HAE expert meeting, training and follow-up is very important both for healthcare staff and patients, especially because self-administration is an option that is increasingly being adopted.

The results of the survey reported by Caballero et al. [2] identified a range of experience worldwide and demonstrated that some healthcare staff request specialist training from personnel in other departments, such as haemophilia and immunology departments. The sharing of expertise is vital to ensure patients are fully trained and are competent in self-administration.

On the practical side of self-administration, as discussed by Symons et al. [3], patients appear to be learning skills quicker than expected and in fewer sessions than guidelines recommend. Nevertheless, the ability to visit patients' homes is restricted in some countries, highlighting the need for potential investment in home care nursing packages. Since home and self-care have evolved differently in different countries, the authors hope that highlighting these differences can stimulate discussion and sharing of ideas leading to improved techniques and education worldwide.

Boysen et al. [4] reported some of the challenges faced by HAE patients and how they have been resolved. One of the main barriers faced by patients being treated in hospital is convincing the treating physician that HAE requires different therapy to the 'usual angioedema'. Moving treatment into the home, especially with self-infusion, removes this barrier and also ensures early therapy. As previously shown, rapid treatment of an HAE attack can markedly reduce time to recovery and morbidity, improves absenteeism and may also be life-saving. More needs to be done to raise awareness of this rare disease and the life-saving implications of rapid treatment.

KARGER

E-Mail karger@karger.com
www.karger.com/iaa

1018–2438/13/1615–0026$38.00/0

Correspondence to: Dr. Timothy J. Craig
College of Medicine, Penn State University
Hershey Medical Center
Hershey, PA 17033 (USA)
E-Mail tcraig@hmc.psu.edu

Table 1. Summary of approved treatments[a]

Drug	Country	Date	Indicated for
Berinert	Germany/Hungary	1979	Acute attacks
	23 EU countries	2008	Acute attacks
	USA	2009	Acute attacks
	Canada	2010	Acute attacks
	23 EU countries	2011	Self-administration for acute attacks
	USA	2012	Self-administration for acute attacks
	23 EU countries	2013	Short-term prophylaxis, including self-administration
Cinryze	USA	2008	Prophylaxis
	USA	2009	Self-administration for prophylaxis
	EU	2011	Acute attacks, routine prevention and short-term prophylaxis, including self-administration
Ruconest	EU	2010	Acute attacks
Icatibant	EU	2008	Acute attacks
	EU	2011	Self-administration for acute attacks
	USA	2011	Self-administration for acute attacks
Ecallantide	USA	2009	Acute attacks

[a] Approvals in countries that participated in the survey.

To aid rapid treatment of an HAE attack, self-administration is a viable treatment option. To make further progress, physicians need to follow their country guidelines more closely, modify them as needed and establish support networks for patients where they are able to seek guidance on care, including self-administration training, effective use of medications, managing their therapy and reporting adverse events.

Self-administration is universally recommended in recent guidelines and in clinical practice. As awareness increases so will the uptake of this treatment option. Although patients are being offered self-administration, not all patients are choosing it and more needs to be done to encourage uptake. The goal of many HAE patients is to be able to manage their own disease and self-administration of therapy can make this desire a reality.

Once again, I would like to express my thanks to all the participants of the international HAE expert meeting for their valuable contributions, and to CSL Behring for their support in the production of this supplement.

Acknowledgements

Editorial assistance was provided by Meridian HealthComms, Plumley, UK, funded by CSL Behring. The survey, international HAE expert meeting and preparation of the supplement were supported by an unrestricted educational grant from CSL Behring.

Notes

Berinert is a registered trademark of CSL Ltd. Group of Companies.

Cinryze is a registered trademark of ViroPharma Biologics Inc.

Firazyr is a registered trademark of Shire and its affiliates.

Kalbitor is a registered trademark of Dyax Corp.

Cetor is a registered trademark of Stichting Sanquin Bloedvoorziening.

Rhucin is a registered trademark of Pharming Group NV.

All trademarks and registered trademarks are the property of their respective owners.

Disclosure Statement

Dr. Craig speaks for CSL Behring, ViroPharma, Shire and Dyax. He does research for Pharming, CSL Behring, ViroPharma, Shire and Dyax. He is a consultant for CSL Behring and Dyax and has received educational grants from Dyax, ViroPharma and CSL Behring.

References

1 Cicardi M, Craig TJ, Martinez-Saguer I, Hébert J, Longhurst HJ: Review of recent guidelines and consensus statements on hereditary angioedema therapy with focus on self-administration. Int Arch Allergy Immunol 2013;161(suppl 1):3–9.

2 Caballero T, Sala-Cunill A, Cancian M, Craig TJ, Neri S, Keith PK, Boccon-Gibod I, Bethune C, Bork K: Current status of implementation of self-administration training in various regions of Europe, Canada and the USA in the management of hereditary angioedema. Int Arch Allergy Immunol 2013; 161(suppl 1):10–16.

3 Symons C, Rossi O, Magerl M, Andritschke K: Practical approach to self-administration of intravenous C1-INH concentrate: a nursing perspective. Int Arch Allergy Immunol 2013; 161(suppl 1):17–20.

4 Boysen HB, Bouillet L, Aygören-Pürsün E: Challenges of C1-inhibitor concentrate self-administration. Int Arch Allergy Immunol 2013;161(suppl 1):21–25.

International Archives of
Allergy and
Immunology

Author Index Vol. 161, Suppl. 1, 2013

Subject Index Vol. 161, Suppl. 1, 2013

KARGER

E-Mail karger@karger.com
www.karger.com/iaa

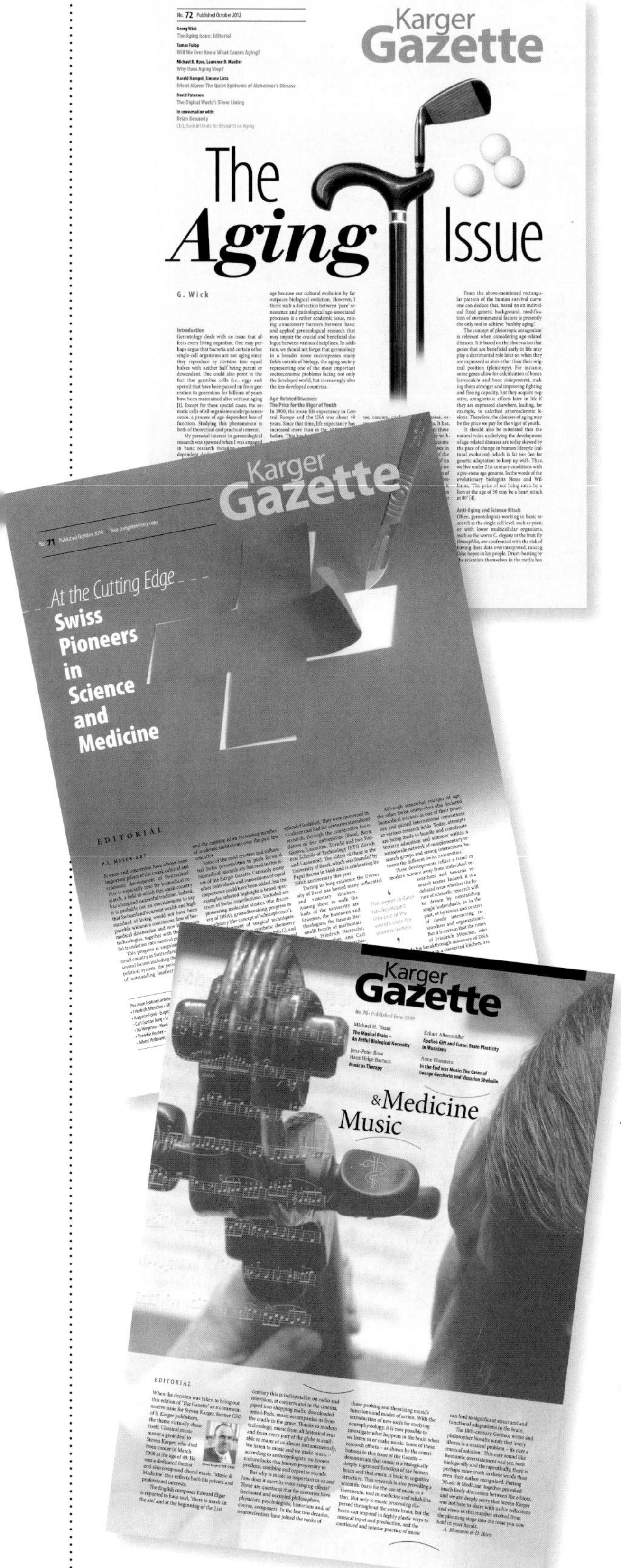

Karger Gazette

Stimulating reading in and around the world of medicine

The biomedical themes of the Karger Gazette are topical, urgent, exciting. Its articles, written by experts from all over the world, provide a wide audience with the basic issues, new findings and controversies in a lively and readable style. Alongside invited contributions, each number carries attractively presented support material, such as informative graphics, historical summaries, interviews, or portraits of individuals and institutions. The Karger Gazette is published in newspaper format and appears once a year.

And what's more – it's free!

To see behind the cover, please write or e-mail us, and we'll start your subscription with the latest issue.

www.karger.com/gazette

Current issue:

The Aging Issue

Read about the causes of the aging process, why aging stops in later adult life, the quiet epidemic of Alzheimer's Disease, internet use by seniors, and more.

S. Karger AG
Karger Gazette
Allschwilerstrasse 10
CH–4009 Basel (Switzerland)
E-Mail gazette@karger.com
www.karger.com

KARGER

KI 12307